D0498016

MURDER

and

MAYHEM

Thomas Dunne Books / St. Martin's Minotaur ≋ New York

MURDER

and

MAYHEM

*A Doctor Answers Medical and
Forensic Questions for Mystery Writers*

D. P. Lyle, M.D.

THOMAS DUNNE BOOKS.
An imprint of St. Martin's Press.

www.minotaurbooks.com

Illustrations by Nan Owen

Library of Congress Cataloging-in-Publication Data

Lyle, D. P.
    Murder & mayhem : a doctor answers medical and forensic questions for
mystery writers / D. P. Lyle.—1st ed.
        p. cm.
    "Thomas Dunne books"—T.p. verso.
    ISBN 0-312-30945-7
    1. Detective and mystery stories—Miscellanea. 2. Forensic sciences—
Miscellanea. I. Title: Murder and mayhem. II. Title.

PN3448.D4 L95 2003
809.3'872—dc21
                                                                2002031887

First Edition: January 2003

10 9 8 7 6 5 4 3 2 1

THIS BOOK IS TO PROVIDE WRITERS OF FICTION WITH ANSWERS TO BASIC AND COMPLEX QUESTIONS ON MEDICAL AND FORENSIC ISSUES. IT IS NOT TO BE USED FOR DIAGNOSIS OR FOR REAL-LIFE BEHAVIOR.

ACKNOWLEDGMENTS

This book would not have been possible without the help of many people. To each I give my sincerest thanks.

My designated readers: Aunt Nancy, Jimmy, Janny, Hawk, Bobbie, Tootie, Sparky, Mikey, Roxy, Stevie B, and Connie.

My patient and friend, Harold Minick, who offered insights from his many years with the Orange County, California, Coroner's Office.

My agent and friend Kimberley Cameron, with Reece Halsey North, and my editor, Sally Kim, of St. Martin's Press/Thomas Dunne Books. Their professionalism, guidance, and enthusiasm throughout the publication process were invaluable.

My parents, Victor and Elaine, who not only gave a lifetime of guidance and support, but also paid for my education.

My sister Vicki, a talented and professional teacher, who taught me to read and write well before my official schooling began.

My sister Melinda for being her life-loving self.

Nan, my better half, who gave me support and allowed me the freedom to pursue the madness of writing, as well as providing the illustrations for this book.

Our feline children, Missy, Peanut, and Bennie, who always make me laugh.

The writers, who, through their questions, constantly amazed me with their dedication to detail and their incredible imaginations.

CONTENTS

4. Medications and Drugs

5. Diseases and Their Treatment

II. *Methods of Murder and Mayhem*

6. The Effects of Guns, Knives, Explosives, and Other Weapons of Death

7. Poisons and Drugs

8. Medical Murder

III. *Tracking the Perp*

9. The Police and the Crime Scene

10. The Coroner, the Crime Lab, and the Autopsy

Odds and Ends, Mostly Odds

A Few Final Words   279

LIST OF ILLUSTRATIONS

MURDER *and* MAYHEM

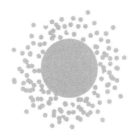

INTRODUCTION

Regardless of genre, every story must possess character and plot. These are the sine qua non of storytelling. Without plot, nothing happens; without character, no one cares what happens. The other story elements—setting, theme, mood, voice, subplots—are solely to support this relationship between protagonist and plot. Thus, a good story is a believable character with which the reader empathizes caught in some life-altering situation.

To reveal character and progress plot, we often place our heroes in stressful situations. Why? Stress brings out the best and the worst in people and makes for interesting and exciting plot elements. There is no better way to stress your protagonist than to apply physical, emotional, and/or psychological pressure.

This is particularly true in the mystery and thriller genres where readers demand to be enthralled, dazzled, informed, and kept awake at night. For this reason mystery and thriller writers often use illness, injury, and psychological stresses such as fear, anxiety, panic, anger, envy, jealousy, remorse, and guilt to thrill and mystify the reader.

In some genres, such as fantasy, allegory, and comedy, the writer can create a world that has no basis in fact or reality. He must, of course, remain true to the rules he has established for that particular world. Short of that restriction, anything is possible.

For mystery and thriller writers the world of their stories is typically "the real world," and therefore "real world" rules must apply.

This places a heavy burden on the writer to get it right. Meticulous research, attention to the smallest detail, and avoidance of a "fast and loose" approach to the facts are essential to building a believable story. Inconsistent motives, convenient resolutions, and errors of fact can undermine even the most likable characters and clever plots.

A major obstacle for many writers is obtaining the specialized knowledge needed to bring their story to life. This is especially true when scientific or medical issues arise. Whether these are the procedures or inner workings of hospitals, emergency departments, or operating rooms; the functioning of doctors, nurses, paramedics, and other paramedical personnel; the mental and physical repercussions of acute or chronic illnesses or injuries such as auto accidents, gunshot wounds, or lightning strikes; the effects of both prescribed and illicit drugs; the impact of acute and chronic psychiatric disorders on victims and their loved ones; or issues in determining the cause and time of death or other forensic procedures, a valid understanding of the complex issues adds depth and drama to any manuscript and lends it the ring of truth.

Where do writers obtain this information? Too often from rehashing the stories of others or echoing what they see on television. Even the promise of the Internet as a source of unlimited information has proven to be false. One can find an overwhelming amount of data on almost every imaginable subject but be ill equipped to separate the truth from the flotsam and jetsam of cyberspace. The old medical adage that "bad data is worse than no data" holds for mystery writing as well.

What This Book Is

This book is intended to inform and entertain not only writers of mysteries and thrillers but also writers in all genres. In addition, lovers of books and movies and anyone with an inquisitive mind will find items of interest within these pages.

This project began at the suggestion of Jan Burke, past president of the Southern California chapter of Mystery Writers of America. She asked if I would write a medical Q and A column for the Southern California chapter's newsletter, *The March of Crime*. My column, "The Doctor Is In," now appears in that publication every month as well as in the newsletter of the Southwestern chapter, *The Sleuth Sayer*.

Since this project began, I have received and attempted to answer hundreds of questions from writers of all genres, including many well-known novelists and screenwriters. Some of the best, most interesting, and most informative are included in this book.

My thanks to each and every writer who submitted a question, for your curiosity, your amazing imagination, and your dedication to "getting it right." I have learned as much from researching and answering your questions as I hope you have from the answers given.

My hope is that all the readers of these pages will find that this material answers some of their questions, raises their level of understanding of medical and forensics issues, causes new questions to germinate, and, most of all, stirs their creative literary juices.

This book is a compilation of some of the medical and forensic questions I have received from writers over the past several years. In the answers I have striven to give writers enough medical and scientific background to provide depth and breadth to their understanding as well as address the nuances of their particular scenario. The goal is to allow writers to use this newly gained understanding to craft more believable scenes or stories. I have attempted to make each question and answer stand alone while minimizing unnecessary repetition of information contained in other questions.

What This Book Is Not

In no way should the material contained in this publication be used for diagnosis or treatment of any medical disorder. Even the simplest question and answer would require decades of education and experience before it could be applied in a real-life situation.

Medicine is an exacting discipline; it is both a science and an art whose mysteries are revealed only after years of practice.

Although I have endeavored to make the information accurate and scientifically correct, many subjects are too complex to explain in detail while addressing the nuances and controversies of modern medical knowledge. Such is the art of medicine. The answers are provided for use in the context of fiction writing and storytelling, and should be used only for such purposes.

This book is not to be used as a manual for any criminal activity or to bring harm to anyone.

Part I

Doctors, Hospitals, Illnesses, and Injuries

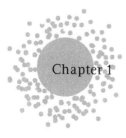

Chapter 1

TRAUMATIC INJURIES AND
THEIR TREATMENT

How Would Death Occur from Blunt Head Trauma?

Q: At the climax of my book there will be a death scene, and I want to make sure I portray it accurately. Essentially, my heroine's love interest sits on a motorcycle that is parked near a curb. The kickstand gives way, and he falls to the side while sitting on the bike. His head hits the curb, the impact killing him. What happens when a person dies from such a head injury? Does blood come out of the ears or nose, or is there no sign of outer trauma? Does the body shake in any way, or will he be found still? At first my heroine doesn't realize that he's hurt. From her view, she can't see the curb. How would he look to her only seconds after he falls? How will he look by the time the paramedics arrive a half hour later?

A: We call this type of injury "blunt trauma," as opposed to "penetrating trauma" from a bullet or axe or other object. Blunt head trauma may result in anything from a simple bump on the head (contusion) to sudden death. The force of the blow alone may cause immediate loss of consciousness (concussion). To cause death, bleeding within or around the brain would most likely have to occur. This is called "intracranial bleeding." It may occur with rupture of an artery, a vein, or multiple small capillaries in and around the brain. Concussions and intracranial bleeds can occur with or without a fracture of the skull.

A membrane called the dura mater covers the brain. The space between the dura and the skull is called the epidural space, while the area between the dura and the brain is termed the subdural space (Figure 1a).

An intracranial bleed is one that occurs anywhere within the skull. They are of three basic types (Figure 1b). Epidural and subdural bleeds occur in the space between the brain and the skull. Epidural bleeds are outside the dura mater and typically result from arterial bleeds from the epidural arteries, which are often torn by fractures of the skull. Subdural bleeds are usually venous in origin and occur in the subdural space. Intracerebral bleeds occur within the brain tissue itself. All are potentially lethal.

Remember, the skull is a rigid capsule that protects the brain. However, if bleeding occurs within the skull or within the brain itself, the bony skull cannot expand. Thus, pressure inside the enclosure rises rapidly, effectively "squeezing" the brain (Figure 1c).

At its posterior (toward the back) base (bottom), the brain narrows into a structure called the brain stem, which narrows further into the spinal cord, which in turn extends along the stack of bones called the spinal column down the back. The brain stem is a vital portion of the brain that, among other things, controls respiration.

The only outlet from the skull cavity is the hole (called the foramen magnum) at the base of the skull where the brain stem and spinal cord exit. It lies near the back juncture of the head and neck. The mounting pressure within the skull shuts down all brain function and ultimately pushes brain material into the foramen magnum and down along the brain stem and spinal cord. Think toothpaste tube. We call this "herniation of the brain stem." Not only is consciousness lost, but the compression of the brain stem also shuts down respiration; death follows in short order.

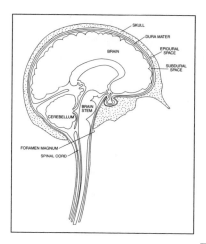

FIGURE IA. THE INTRACRANIAL SPACES
The dura mater is a protective membrane that surrounds the brain. The space above the dura is the epidural space ("epi" means above) and the space beneath is the subdural space ("sub" means below). Bleeding can occur in either area.

FIGURE IB. THE THREE BASIC TYPES OF INTRACRANIAL BLEEDS
All bleeds within the skull (cranium) are called intracranial bleeds. Those that occur within the brain tissue itself are intracerebral bleeds. Bleeding in the area around the brain may be either epidural or subdural, depending on the exact location of the bleed.

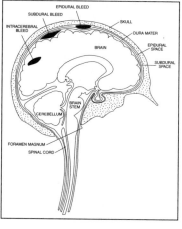

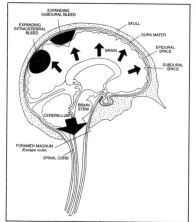

FIGURE IC. MECHANISM OF BRAIN STEM HERNIATION
Bleeding in or around the brain causes a rapid elevation of pressure within the rigid skull. The only escape route for this excess pressure is through the foramen magnum, an opening at the base of the skull through which the brain stem and spinal cord exit. The extrusion or "herniation" of brain material through this opening compresses the brain stem, resulting in cessation of respiration and then death.

This process may occur over minutes, hours, or days. Remember how when you hit your head as a kid your mother would check you throughout the night to see if you were okay? That's because the bleeding may be slow, and headaches and coma and death may not occur for several hours. See, Mom was right.

Occasionally, people who have suffered blunt trauma do not develop any neurologic symptoms until days or weeks later. When headaches, nausea, blurred vision, numbness, or weakness in their extremities (all symptoms associated with rising intracranial pressure) occur, they visit a doctor, and a slow intracranial bleed is discovered.

The most likely injury in your situation would be a skull fracture with a rupture or tearing of an epidural artery (one of the many small arteries that course over the surface of the brain and are often torn with skull fractures), which would lead to bleeding. This would be classified as an epidural bleed. Arterial bleeding is usually brisk, and rising intracranial pressure, coma, apnea (loss of respiration), and death can occur very rapidly.

Most likely your victim would merely lie there, neither moving nor breathing. Such trauma could trigger seizure activity, though usually not, and that wouldn't fit your scenario anyway. When the heroine sees him immediately after the event, he may appear as if he is merely asleep. With a skull fracture a trickle of blood may appear from the ear or nose or both. Also, he may have a blue-black swelling (contusion) at the point of impact. Or there may be no external signs of injury.

A half hour later he would look . . . dead: blue-gray skin, flaccid (limp) limbs, dilated black pupils, no breathing, no pulse. The paramedics would most likely institute CPR and transport the victim to a hospital, where an M.D. would make the death pronouncement.

Can My Heroine Survive an Auto Accident and Ruptured Spleen?

Q: My sleuth is forced at gunpoint to drive to a remote area where she is certain she will be murdered. Her kidnapper, another woman, is riding in the passenger seat. They are traveling on a road temporarily closed for resurfacing. As they pass a few pieces of parked road equipment, my sleuth, desperate to save herself, spots a heavy-equipment trailer and veers into it at 30 miles per hour, hoping to selectively destroy the passenger side of the car. The steel trailer's rear bumper peels away the car's roof like the lid from a can, decapitating her tormentor. My heroine survives but is trapped with both shoulders broken and waits a half hour before being rescued. Later at the hospital we learn she has an injured spleen and is teetering between life and death. Needless to say, she is alive and beginning her long recovery by morning. Is my explanation way off the mark?

A: A ruptured spleen fits this scenario perfectly. Blunt trauma in a car accident, which is likely from a steering wheel injury, often results in a splenic rupture. It is very common in motorcycle accidents, football and skateboarding injuries, and so forth.

The spleen is a vascular organ (has a lot of blood in it); it sits in the left upper abdomen, tucked behind the lower margins of the ribs (Figure 2). It receives its blood from the splenic artery, a fairly large blood vessel. The spleen has a thin capsule that encases the soft and spongy splenic tissue (think blood-soaked sponge); thus it can rupture like a melon. In fact, its capsule is very easy to rupture or tear, and when breached, it will bleed profusely. During abdominal surgical procedures the spleen is handled with great care

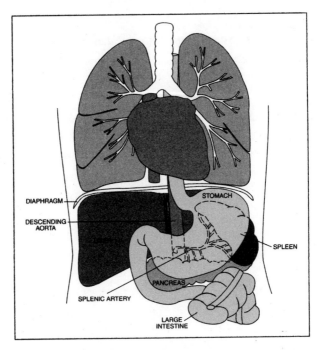

FIGURE 2. THE SPLEEN
The spleen lies in the upper left corner of the abdomen, tucked
behind the lower edge of the rib cage. It is easily damaged by blunt
abdominal trauma such as occurs in automobile accidents or falls.

because even the delicate manipulations of the surgeon's fingers
can injure it.

Although they can, people don't usually die from splenic ruptures. The reason? After enough blood is lost, the blood pressure
(BP) drops, and the flow of blood into the splenic artery and the
spleen lessens, the bleeding slows, and the process stops. The blood
pressure of the injured person may go down to 60 or 70, but he or
she can survive for a while in this degree of shock. The classic
example of a splenic rupture is the teenager who slams his motor-
bike into a tree or car and arrives at the ER awake but lethargic
with a BP of 70. Interestingly, once the victim is given blood and
fluids and the BP begins to rise, the bleeding worsens—higher BP,

more blood into the spleen, more bleeding. Emergency surgery is the definitive treatment.

Of course, with your character stuck in the sitting position, gravity will hasten and magnify the degree of BP drop and the resulting shock syndrome. Still, she should survive the incident unless medical care is delayed too long.

Your character could exhibit several different symptoms as she waits for help and slips deeper into shock. Besides the pain in her damaged shoulders and abdomen, as the BP drops and shock sets in, your character will develop some or all of the following symptoms: dizziness, confusion, disorientation, hallucinations, nausea, vomiting, chills, shivering, thirst, cold sweats, blurred vision, sleepiness, weakness, a heavy feeling in her neck and extremities, and, finally, sleep or coma. Her reflection in the rearview mirror would be pale, even ghostly white, and maybe with a cyanotic tint (blue-gray hue due to shock and low blood oxygen levels). She may be in and out of consciousness or perhaps have vivid remembrances of things past akin to waking dreams.

Once rescued she will need immediate IV fluids, blood, and surgery to remove the spleen (splenectomy). Injured spleens are rarely repaired and almost always removed, since the spongy nature of the splenic tissue makes it very difficult to "fix." Besides, the spleen is not a vital organ, and people tend to get along quite well without one.

She should recover completely from the splenic rupture and splenectomy, and were this her only injury, she would be out of bed in a couple of days, home in a week, and back to normal by six weeks. However, recovery from her shoulder injuries, which could require surgical repair, would take a few months. The shoulder surgery would likely be delayed for several days after the splenectomy so she could be stabilized and prepared for this procedure. Before and after the surgery, the shoulders would be immobilized by placing her arms in slings, and she would require sedation and analgesic medications for the pain.

Where Can My Hero Be Shot and Survive?

Q: In my story the protagonist is shot. Obviously, he survives, but he is partially incapacitated. He must overcome the antagonist in a hand-to-hand fight. Where could he be shot and still function?

A: First, let's look at what happens when someone suffers a gunshot wound (GSW in medical shorthand). Ask any emergency department physician, and he will tell you that killing someone with a gun is not that easy. For a GSW to be immediately lethal, it must disrupt brain and/or heart function. Thus, a direct shot to the brain or heart is usually deadly in very short order. Also, a GSW to the lungs or a major blood vessel, such as the aorta, could be lethal in a manner of minutes or hours. Additionally, GSWs to the head, chest, or abdomen are severely incapacitating and would probably not fit your story.

That said, I might point out the following:

Many GSWs to the head do not penetrate the skull and thus do little brain damage. If the bullet approaches from a shallow angle, it may bounce off the skull and exit into the air or burrow beneath the scalp. In this situation a GSW that appears to be deadly at first would cause little harm, and your protagonist would fight on.

A GSW to the chest likewise might not penetrate the chest cavity, but instead might glance off a rib or the sternum (breastbone). In this case no major organ damage would occur, and your hero could continue his pursuit. The bullet might fracture a rib, which would be very painful with any movement and with breathing, particularly if he has to chase the villain.

A GSW to the abdomen might be well tolerated by your hero even if it doesn't simply embed in the flesh or muscles of the abdominal wall (which frequently happens) and actually penetrates the abdominal cavity. It would be very painful, more so than a GSW almost anywhere else, because the internal abdominal lining (peritoneum) is loaded with nerve fibers. But if no major blood vessel or organ (liver, kidney, or spleen) is damaged, your protagonist, if he is tough, could fight through the pain and overcome the enemy. Think James Bond.

A GSW to an extremity seems best for your scenario. This would slow down your hero, but again, unless a major blood vessel was breached, it would not kill or greatly maim him. Besides, the injury could be tailored to hamper your hero's efforts to the greatest degree. If he must chase down the villain, then shoot him in the leg or hip or foot. If he must climb a rope or ladder or wrestle with the antagonist, shoot him in the arm. If he must swim, have the bullet enter his shoulder.

I should also point out that people who suffer severe and potentially lethal GSWs often live long enough to kill their attacker or crawl to a phone or scrawl the killer's name in their own blood. If your protagonist is shot during the climax of your story, the wound could be more serious because he could survive long enough to do in the villain, call for medical help, and heal before the sequel.

Can a Person with Broken Ribs Swim?

Q: One of my characters is hit in the chest while standing on a sailboat and is knocked overboard. I later say that the blow broke a couple of ribs and one of the ribs punctured a lung, causing it to collapse. Using one arm he manages to keep himself afloat for the three or four minutes it takes for someone to haul him back aboard, using the boat's emergency sling.

Would a person with a broken rib, let alone a collapsed lung, be able to use his arm well enough to keep himself afloat? And assuming that this character received competent medical treatment in a modern hospital within two hours of the accident, how long would it be before he could plausibly make his next appearance in the story?

A: A rib fracture is extremely painful, especially since we can't "rest" it or immobilize it while it heals. A broken arm is splinted or placed in a cast; the chest cannot be restricted in this fashion, since breathing is not optional.

Inhaling air into the lungs is an active process. The muscles between the ribs work to expand the chest, creating the negative pressure within the chest cavity required to pull air into the lungs. A fractured rib makes this an extremely painful process.

The pain is typically localized to the area of the fracture and is very sharp—like a knife sticking into the chest. Each breath is excruciating. We call this type of pain "pleuritic." It results not only from the broken rib itself but also from the highly enervated (has a lot of nerves) lining of the chest cavity, called the "pleura."

If the sharp end of the broken rib protrudes into the chest cavity, it may puncture the lung, causing it to collapse. We call this a "pneumothorax." The pneumo (for short) may be small or large, meaning the degree of lung collapse may be minor or significant. We grade these by percentage of collapse. A minor pneumothorax would be 10 to 20 percent, while a large pneumo would be 50 percent or more. A complete collapse would of course be a 100 percent pneumo.

A minor collapse is painful but otherwise not severely debilitating. A complete collapse is painful and associated with marked shortness of breath. It would be lethal only if the victim has significant underlying heart or lung disease or if the pneumo is of the "tension" type. In a tension pneumothorax the hole in the lung acts as a ball valve, or one-way leak (Figure 3a). When the victim inhales, air passes from the lung, through the hole, and into the

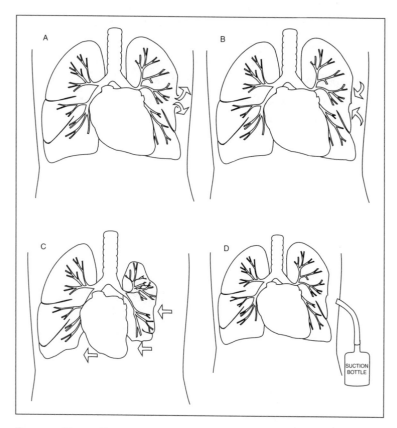

FIGURE 3. TENSION PNEUMOTHORAX
The development of a tension pneumothorax requires that the puncture site act as a one-way valve. During inhalation, air can pass from the lung into the chest cavity (3a); during exhalation, the one-way valve blocks egress of the air, thus trapping it in the chest cavity (3b). As the air accumulates, pressure rises within the chest and compresses the heart and the contralateral "good" lung (3c). Successful treatment requires the placement of a thoracostomy (chest) tube into the chest cavity and the removal of the air by use of a suction device (3d). This allows the lung to re-expand and heal.

chest cavity (Figure 3a), yet when he attempts to exhale, the air cannot pass back through the hole, into the lung, and out through the mouth (Figure 3b). Each breath increases pressure within the chest, collapsing the lung further. As the pressure (tension) mounts, the heart and the "good" lung also become compressed, resulting in declining heart and lung function and ultimately death (Figure

3c). This may occur rapidly, over minutes. Fortunately, most pneumos are not of the tension variety.

Long-term treatment also depends on the degree of collapse. With minor pneumos, the victim is often observed in the hospital for a few days. The leak usually seals itself, the lung reinflates, and the person goes home and experiences a few weeks of chest pain as the fracture heals. When it is a major collapse, a thoracostomy tube (or chest tube) is inserted (Figure 3d). This plastic tube goes through the chest wall and into the chest cavity between the chest wall and the lung. Suction is applied for several days, allowing the lung to reinflate and the leak to heal. The tube is then removed. Subsequent recovery is the same as with a minor leak but may take a couple of weeks longer.

In your scenario a fracture with a minor pneumo would work. Yes, he could swim. Yes, he could fight if necessary. Yes, it would be very painful, but heroes are forged from pain and perseverance. He could return to action in a few days if absolutely necessary or if he is stubborn and not one to follow doctor's orders.

What Is the Mechanism of Death in a Suicide by Hanging?

Q: A man in my novel commits suicide by tying a rope around his neck and kicking a step stool away. He's discovered about half an hour later. Is the cause of death, then, strangulation? Would he have urinated or defecated in the course of dying? Would there be a smell? Also, what would his face look like? Would he have died differently if there was a drop of six feet? Can I assume a different cause of death? Broken neck? Would his face look different? Would his neck be distorted in any way?

A: The result of a hanging depends on several factors—the weight of the victim, the size and muscularity of his neck, and the distance of the drop, to name a few. If the victim drops several feet, the noose would indeed fracture his neck, and death would be fairly instantaneous. He would simply fall and then hang limply. Yes, he would likely evacuate his bladder and bowels, and the smell would be as expected.

On the other hand, if the fall is short, as in kicking a chair or stool out of the way or having a horse spooked from beneath him—a staple in old Westerns—his neck would not break, and death would be from strangulation. It would be slow and painful, with a great deal of kicking and struggling. When death finally occurs, the victim would likely soil himself as above.

In the latter case, his face would be purplish and engorged with blood. His eyes would protrude; perhaps his tongue would be swollen and protruding; and his neck would be excoriated from the struggle against the rope. Also, the conjunctivae—the pink part of the inside of the eyelid—would show petechial hemorrhages. These look like small bright red spots, and they result from the increased pressure in the veins and capillaries in the tender tissues. Similar findings are common in manual or ligature strangulations.

Most suicides by hanging are poorly executed and the victim does not fracture his neck and thus dies from asphyxiation or strangulation. When the chair is gone and the person finds that he isn't dead, religion and panic take over in short order, and a life-and-death struggle ensues, regardless of how committed the person was to the suicide in the first place. Suddenly, what looked good on paper isn't so attractive. And since in self-hangings the victim usually cannot tie his hands behind his back, he will use them in his struggles for survival. He will claw at his neck or try to climb the rope to ease the pressure of the noose. This results in scratches and tears of the flesh, ripping loose of fingernails, and rope burns on palms and fingers.

What Wounds Would Result from an Attempted Suicide with a Gun Placed Under the Chin?

Q: If a character commits suicide by firing a handgun placed under his chin, and the gun is loaded with "hot loads" (overpowered magnum rounds intended for use against vehicles and similar targets), what kind of ballistic results could be expected? Would the resulting injury produce a relatively small hole due to overpenetration, or would the mushrooming effect obliterate most of the skull; in other words, is there sufficient resistance to the bullet to cause it to mushroom? Is there a chance of survival, or is this technique highly effective? Aside from "gray matter," is there likely to be much blood?

A: Yes, this is effective and virtually 100 percent fatal provided the gun doesn't slip and the angle change. I saw a man years ago who placed a shotgun under his chin and pulled the trigger. He had angled the barrel slightly forward and opened his face as if someone had cleaved it with an axe. The shot never entered the skull and he was neurologically intact and awake when the paramedics arrived. A plastic surgeon and a neurosurgeon put him back together. But short of such an odd occurrence, this type of approach is uniformly fatal.

Typically, the entry wound is relatively small and the exit wound large, likely removing the entire skullcap and most of the brain. There would be a great deal of tissue and blood. However, a bullet coated with Teflon or otherwise manufactured to "penetrate armor" probably would not "mushroom," and therefore both entry and exit wounds would be small and there would be less tissue and blood. Still effective, but less messy.

Can a Traumatic Miscarriage Prevent Future Pregnancies?

Q: I have a character who is three months pregnant. She is injured in an automobile accident and suffers a miscarriage. Later the doctor tells her she can never have children again. Is this possible? What would have to happen to her to make future pregnancies impossible?

A: Yes, your scenario is possible.

First, let's deal with the accident and the miscarriage. Blunt trauma to the abdomen as occurs in auto accidents (AA) can result in miscarriage. In AAs the seat belt itself can injure the lower abdomen and thus the uterus. If no seat belt is worn, collisions with the steering wheel, dashboard, or seat back (if she is sitting in the backseat) can result in similar injuries. Falls down stairs (a Hollywood staple for this scenario) and kicks or punches, as can occur in domestic abuse situations, can lead to similar injuries.

During pregnancy the fetus floats inside the uterus in amniotic fluid, which serves as some protection from trauma. But if enough force is applied, the fetus can be injured or killed. Or the placenta that nourishes the fetus and is attached to the inner wall of the uterus can be torn loose. Bleeding into the uterine cavity or loss of placental support for the fetus can result in fetal death and miscarriage. In severe trauma the uterus can rupture, and the fetus and even the mother can be lost. As the uterus expands during pregnancy, its walls thin, and it becomes increasingly prone to this catastrophe with each passing month.

If the uterus is intact but the fetus is no longer viable, a dilatation and curettage (D and C) must be done to remove the dead fetus and placenta. Dilatation means the dilating or opening up of the cervix, which the surgeon must do to reach the inside of the uterus. Curettage is the removal of material from the walls of a cavity—in this case the fetus and placenta from the uterus. If the uterus ruptures, a true medical emergency exists, and surgery must be performed immediately to save the mother. Often the uterus must be removed under these circumstances, though at times it can be repaired and salvaged.

To make future pregnancy impossible, either the uterus itself or its delicate lining would have to be damaged to the point that implantation (the attachment of the fertilized egg to the uterine lining) can no longer occur. Or the uterus could be scarred in such a manner that even if implantation does occur, the uterus cannot support fetal growth and development. After trauma and a D and C, either of these is a possible outcome. Obviously, if the uterus is removed (hysterectomy), pregnancy is precluded.

If your character suffers a uterine rupture in the AA, she would have severe lower abdominal pain and vaginal bleeding, and it is likely she would go into shock: She would be pale, cold, sweaty, delirious, or unconscious, and have a very weak pulse and low blood pressure. The paramedics would begin IVs, give lots of fluids such as D5LR (5 percent dextrose in lactated Ringer's solution), administer oxygen, and speed to the nearest hospital or trauma unit. She would be taken to surgery almost immediately for an emergency hysterectomy. Recovery, if all went well, would take five to seven days in the hospital and then six to eight weeks at home. Of course, the tremendous psychological stress this would cause might take years to overcome.

What Are the Symptoms of a Concussion?

Q: If my character is struck on the head with an object and knocked unconscious for ten or fifteen minutes, what symptoms will he have when he wakes up? Amnesia? How long will these symptoms last?

A: In medical terms, this is called a concussion. It is a transient loss of consciousness or alteration of consciousness (dazed) associated with some degree of amnesia. This typically occurs in blunt trauma to the head as you describe or in deceleration injuries that occur in auto accidents, falls, and so forth.

The mechanism of the loss of consciousness appears to be a disruption of the electrophysiologic function of the reticular activation system (RAS). This is an area at the base of the brain that is responsible for maintaining consciousness. The blow seems to scramble its electrical circuits for a while, resulting in loss of consciousness. The mechanism of the amnesia is unclear.

The symptoms associated with such injuries vary, but headache, dizziness, and amnesia are common. Lethargy and confusion are less common. Ringing in the ears and blurred or double vision are even less common. Also uncommon are seizures.

These symptoms may last a few minutes, hours, or days. In some people they may last for weeks or months. Professional football quarterbacks and boxers seem particularly prone to concussions. Steve Young and Troy Aikman each missed from one to several weeks of football after their many concussions because their symptoms—mostly dizziness and headache—lasted that long. A knockout (KO) in a boxing match is simply a concussion.

The amnesia may be just for the period of unconsciousness, may continue for a short while after the injury, or may be retrograde so that the victim doesn't remember things that occurred prior to the injury. For example, people who suffer concussions in auto accidents may not remember getting in the car, leaving home, or where they were going.

If the victim suffers a seizure after the blow, a complete neurologic evaluation should be undertaken to rule out the presence of damage to or bleeding into or around the brain. Skull and neck X rays, CT scans or MRIs, and hospital admission for observation are recommended in this situation.

The treatment for an uncomplicated concussion is time and the avoidance of any further trauma. For headache, Tylenol, aspirin, Darvocet, or Vicodin may be prescribed as well as other analgesics (pain relievers). For dizziness, Dramamine, Meclizine, and Antivert are often used. These are the same medications used for motion sickness. Typically, the victim returns to normal in a few minutes, a few hours, or a few days.

What Happens When You Get the "Wind Knocked Out of You"?

Q: My character suffers a blow to the stomach and gets the wind knocked out of her. What really happens? How long will it take her to recover?

A: When someone receives a severe blunt force injury to the solar plexus—the area of the abdomen between the lower end of the sternum (breastbone) and the umbilicus (belly button)—she actually stops breathing for a few seconds. Many of the nerves that leave the spinal cord and spread out to all parts of the body pass through relay stations called "ganglia" (the singular is ganglion). Several of these ganglia lie behind the stomach, near the aorta. The major ones are the celiac ganglion and the superior and inferior mesenteric ganglia. Together they are often referred to as the solar plexus.

A sharp blow to this area causes these ganglia and nerves to release massive and erratic impulses for a few seconds. This in turn causes the diaphragm to spasm, or cramp. The diaphragm is a muscular partition between the chest and the abdomen, and its movement draws air into the lungs and forces it out of the lungs. When it spasms, the person cannot breathe, and thus the wind is knocked out of them.

The symptoms are pain (from the blow and from the spasm of the diaphragm—think leg cramp or charley horse)—and the feeling of smothering from the inability to breathe. Often the person's eyes will water, she will bend over or drop to the ground, and she will try to take in air, which can't occur until the diaphragm relaxes and returns to normal function. Fear plays a great role here, because the person feels as if she may never be able to breathe again.

Fortunately, within a few seconds (five to twenty or so), the nervous system regroups, the diaphragm relaxes, and breathing resumes. These few seconds are, of course, an eternity for the one who can't breathe. After that it takes a few minutes for the victim to recover completely, and then she would be able to do anything. She may experience mild residual soreness from the blow and the diaphragmatic spasm, but overall she would be normal and have no long-term injury.

What Injuries Occur When Someone Is Thrown Down a Stairway?

Q: My protagonist tosses two twenty-something hoods down a short set of concrete steps. Following this encounter, for plot purposes I need each hood to be physically incapable of pursuing my protagonist for different lengths of time—one for several days, and the other for a full week or so. The former must be conscious during his period of incapacitation or hospitalization, but not necessarily the latter. Additionally, the former must recover to the point where he can still do my protagonist serious bodily harm should the two meet again. Can you offer some suggestions for the type of injuries the two hoods could suffer and meet my plot criteria?

A: A tumble down stairs offers several realistic opportunities for injury. Either of your hoods could suffer any of the traumas I'll detail, the difference being severity.

Fractures

Concrete stairs can fracture bones—arms, legs, shoulders, hips, ribs, and skulls. Any of these could prevent the hoods from immediately chasing the hero, particularly skull, leg, and hip fractures. Each of these would require several weeks for full recovery.

Hip: A hip fracture would require surgery and the hood would be laid up for months. He would be conscious after his fall but wouldn't be able to chase your hero for at least four to six months.

Skull: With a skull fracture the victim could be conscious or out for minutes to several days. Your choice. Recovery would be a couple of months, and while it wouldn't be advisable for him to fight anyone, he could. In fact, if he were a tough guy, he might be able to fight in a few days. Hell of a headache, but possible. I doubt most readers would buy this, though. A skull fracture might work for hood number two.

Leg: A fractured femur (upper leg) is similar to a hip fracture and would require surgery and months of recuperation. A fracture of either the tibia or fibula (lower leg bones) may or may not require surgery but would require a cast for four to six weeks.

Shoulder: Fractured shoulders often need surgery, but if the shoulder joint is only dislocated, probably not. He would be out of action for several weeks if surgery was required but only a day or two if dislocated. However, he would be in considerable pain and would be "one-armed," if that works for you. In shoulder separations or dislocations the arm is typically strapped against the body for a few weeks until the torn and strained ligaments heal.

Arm: A fracture of the humerus (the upper arm) is a similar situation to a shoulder fracture. A fracture of the radius or ulna (lower arm bones) would require a cast for several weeks. The victim would be left to fight with only one arm, though a cast makes a great weapon.

Rib: Assuming the fractured rib didn't puncture the lung, he would be very sore for a few days and fairly sore for a few weeks. He could renew his pursuit of the hero after several days. This might work for hood number one. The pain from a fractured rib can be severe and is usually sharp and stabbing; it is made worse with breathing and movement of the shoulders or chest. The villain could fight but would be in considerable pain.

If the rib punctured and collapsed the lung, his hospitalization and recovery would be longer and more complicated.

Head Trauma

A concussion would work well since the victim would be "out" for minutes to hours and then would be okay except for a residual headache. Other residual symptoms might be dizziness, mild nausea, blurred vision, and a stiff neck. These could be mild or severe, and could last for a day or two or up to several weeks. The victim could return to battle in a day or several days if you wish. Either works medically. Think NFL quarterback.

Muscular Strains

A muscular strain of the back, especially the lower back, would make immediate pursuit impossible but would likely abate after several days of treatment with pain medications and muscle relaxants. Then he would be able to attack the hero with little limitation. Or he could have continued pain and stiffness, which would hamper his ability to pursue and fight.

Internal Injuries

A fall down concrete steps is similar to an automobile accident. All sorts of internal injuries could occur. Lacerated livers, ruptured spleens, and fractured kidneys would require surgery and a prolonged recovery. A contused (bruised) kidney might work for you. Here the trauma of the fall bruises the kidney, causing flank pain and bloody urine. Recovery would be a few days to a few weeks, after which he could chase and fight with your hero. A little sore, but functional.

Hood number one could have a muscular strain, concussion, rib fracture, or contused kidney, and would not be unconscious during recovery and would be able to fight again in a few days.

Hood number two could have more serious fractures (hip, leg, shoulder, skull) or a more severe concussion (even with a bleed into the brain), a rib fracture with or without a punctured lung, or internal injuries. He could be in a coma for almost any period of time, or he could be awake throughout. His recovery could take weeks to months.

What Injuries Occur in a Fall onto Rocks?

Q: For my story, I need to know what general or specific damage might a man incur if he is shoved off a cliff, falls 60 feet, and lands on craggy rocks. Is a 60-foot drop long enough to guarantee death?

A: A 60-foot fall onto craggy rocks is universally fatal unless a semi-miracle occurs. People have jumped from planes with parachute failure and lived to tell about it. These cases are extremely rare, however, and the people usually land in a recently plowed field or something equally as forgiving. Needless to say, this is not a common occurrence.

The fall would break arms and legs and skulls and spines; mush kidneys and livers and lungs and spleens; and rupture stomachs and colons and bladders and aortas. A mess, to say the least.

With this type of fall you generally have carte blanche regarding the types of injuries you want the victim to suffer as long as they are severe. There are no minor injuries in this situation.

If the body is discovered during the period of rigor mortis rigidity, it will be stiff and "frozen" in the position the victim was in at the time of death. Remember, rigor comes on during the first twelve hours and then resolves over the next twenty-four. If the body is discovered before or after that general time frame, it would be limp, and when the victim is lifted, the bones might crunch and grind as if he were a bag of marbles.

Of course, many of the fractures might be compound, meaning the broken bones puncture the skin, and the abdomen or chest may have ruptured. Also, the craggy rocks may cause lacerations and deep tears in the tissues of the arms, legs, abdomen, and chest, or they may penetrate the skull directly rather than the skull's being fractured from the impact. Not pretty.

What Is the Likely Cause of Death in a Fall Downstairs?

Q: Is it possible for a female character, age thirty-four, to fall down a flight of fourteen exterior steps and die? She is drinking heavily all night and wearing five-inch spike heels. Is there anything special she would need to fall on? What would cause death? I thought she could hit her head, but do you have any other thoughts? If someone shoved her, would there be any way to tell during an autopsy?

A: This type of death happens every day, especially to people "under the influence." Steps, ladders, and bathtubs are the most dangerous places in the average house. A fall down fourteen steps could result in severe and deadly injuries, and in many ways it is similar to an automobile accident.

Death can result from many different injuries. Rupture of the liver, spleen, or another internal organ can lead to internal bleeding and death. A fracture of the femur (the upper leg bone) would be a likely injury and could also be lethal. When the femur is shattered, its sharp edges can lacerate the large arteries and veins of the leg, and massive blood loss and death can follow. If the bone punches through the skin (a "compound fracture"), bleeding would be through the puncture and out of the body. But even if a compound doesn't occur and the skin remains unbroken, massive and lethal bleeding can still occur. The thigh can hold a few quarts of blood, which may be enough to cause shock and death.

However, a head or neck injury would be best. Either a broken neck or an intracranial bleed, which is bleeding in and around the brain with or without a fracture of the skull, would fit your scenario well. Death can be instantaneous or may take minutes, hours, or even days.

A shove would not likely leave any marks that the coroner could identify. At autopsy the M.E. would find an intoxicated woman with either a neck fracture or a bleed into the brain, and could easily conclude the death was accidental.

What Happens When Someone's Nose Is Broken?

Q: What does a guy look like after a broken nose? Does it have to be operated on? Is it possible to suffer a severe blow to the nose and just have a nosebleed and no fracture?

A: The victim's nose could simply bleed; or it could swell up, turn purple, and bleed; or it could be shattered and deformed, even flattened, and bleed. Regardless, it would bleed. Since the inside lining of the nose (called the "nasal mucosa") is very vascular, bleeding is common even in minor injuries.

The nose is mostly cartilage; only its base is bone. Since the cartilage is flexible and springy, sometimes a heavy blow only damages the soft tissues and no fracture occurs. Sometimes the cartilage or the bone, or both, will fracture. Anything is possible.

A fractured nose is often maneuvered back to its original position, bandaged, and allowed to heal. Though it usually isn't, surgery may be required. Often a short metal splint is taped along the nose to support it during the healing phase.

The injured nose would remain black and blue—as would the area beneath the eyes, since the blood tends to collect there—for at least two weeks.

How Long Will a Black Eye Persist?

Q: My character gets punched in the face, near her eye. How long will her black eye last?

A: Bruises (contusions) are caused by the leakage of blood from the small capillary blood vessels that have been injured due to some trauma. A fist in the eye, a thigh banged against a table corner, and a twist of an ankle are traumas that can lead to bruising. The extent of the resulting blue-black discoloration depends on how much blood seeps from the damaged vessels, and it varies in different areas of the body. The tissues around the eyes (the periorbital area) are very vascular (loaded with blood vessels) and soft. As a result, they bruise easily and severely. The discoloration that appears in this area is much more pronounced and more prolonged than a contusion of the thigh or the arm. In periorbital contusions the effect of gravity often pulls the blood, and thus the bruise, downward into the upper cheek.

The seepage of blood from the capillaries continues over two to three days, so the bruise expands and darkens during this phase. That is why you should apply ice to contusions for the first seventy-two hours. It helps the blood clot by slowing its flow, which reduces the leak and thus lessens the bruising.

From day three to about day ten the blood that has leaked into the tissues is broken down and removed by the body's enzymes and scavenger cells (macrophages). The initial deep blue-black color progressively fades.

From day ten through about day twenty the purplish remnant of the bruise becomes brownish green and/or brownish yellow. This is due to the body's enzymatic destruction of hemoglobin (the iron-containing oxygen-carrying molecule in the red blood cells), which produces breakdown products that possess these characteristic colors. These, in turn, are consumed and carried away by the macrophages. The discoloration should resolve by day twenty, and the skin color in the contused area should return to normal.

In summary, the blue-black bruise deepens and expands over three days, lightens and begins to fade over the next seven days, changes to a brownish, yellowish, then greenish color, continues to fade over the next ten days, and finally resolves.

Your character should be able to cover the damage with makeup after day seven to ten or so.

Where Would the Spinal Cord Have to Be Injured to Cause Quadriplegia?

Q: A character in my story is paralyzed when he walks away from a confrontation and is shot in the back. He becomes a quadriplegic with some use of his right arm and hand, and he can breathe without help from a respirator. Where would the bullet enter the spinal cord to cause this? What caliber bullet would be required?

A: The spinal cord extends from the brain stem, which protrudes from the base of the brain, down the back. It is protected by the bones of the spinal column. Along its path the cord sends nerves out to the lungs, heart, arms, legs, and so forth. Think of the spinal cord as the main electrical cable into your house. As it extends from one room to the next, it splits off branches to the living room, bedroom, kitchen, garage, and so forth. If the main cable is severed, the branches that come off after the area of damage will fail, while those that split off earlier will continue to function. In the above sequence, if the cable is cut between the bedroom and the kitchen, the kitchen appliances will no longer work and the garage door opener will be dead. The lights in the living room and bedroom would not be affected. Similarly, if the spinal cord is damaged, all the body parts distal (downstream) of the area of damage will cease to function properly.

Functionally, the spinal cord is divided into "levels," though if you viewed it anatomically, it would show no such divisions. The spinal cord levels are named to correspond with the spinal vertebra at any given level. The major levels are the cervical (neck), thoracic (chest), lumbar (lower back), and sacral (tail or buttocks). There are eight cervical vertebra and cord levels designated C1 through C8; twelve thoracic (T1 through T12); five lumbar (L1 through L5); and five sacral (S1 through S5).

Each level sends its nerves out to different parts of the body. These areas of enervation are called "dermatomes," and charts exist that show what level of the cord sends nerves to what parts of the body (Figure 4). When a physician examines a patient with a spinal injury, he can determine the level of the injury by determining what parts of the body have defective motor (movement) or sensory (sensation) functions. For example, C2 enervates the scalp and jaw, T10 the body at the level of the umbilicus (belly button), and L1 through L3 the upper legs. If the physician finds that no cord function exists below the level of the umbilicus, he may con-

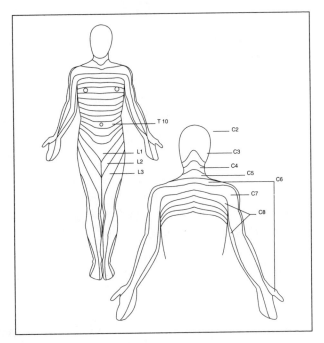

FIGURE 4. THE DERMATOMES OF THE BODY
The nervous system of the human body is intricate but orderly. Each neurologic level is predictable and helps in determining the location of injuries to the spinal cord.

clude that the cord was injured at about T10. In this case the victim would be deemed paraplegic, since he would have lost use of his lower extremities while everything above T10 would function normally.

In your scenario the important levels would be C3 though C5, which control the diaphragm and respiration, and C6 through C8, which enervate the upper extremities. Your character's injury must be below C5 for respiration to be intact but above C8 if most of his upper extremity function is lost. This means that an injury at the C6 or C7 level would work. This corresponds to a bullet entry wound near where the neck joins the shoulders in back. An injury at this level would allow the victim to retain the ability to breathe while losing function of one or both arms.

It is important to note that the defect doesn't have to be symmetric; that is, the left side can be affected more than the right, and vice versa. So your character could have some or even complete use of his right arm and hand, and complete paralysis of the left. Such is the nature of these types of injuries.

Any gun could cause this injury. Small calibers, such as .22 and .32, could sever the cord with a direct hit. Larger calibers, such as .357 and .44, can do a lot more damage and injure the cord with a less-than-direct hit.

Could My Pregnant Character and Her Unborn Child Survive a Severe Concussion and Near Drowning?

Q: One of my characters is a woman who is six months pregnant. During an explosion she bashes her head on an indoor swimming pool ladder and falls unconscious into the pool. She is without oxygen for an undetermined amount of time, but not long. Mouth-to-mouth is performed almost immediately, and she begins to breathe but doesn't regain consciousness. At the hospital the doctor determines that she is in a light coma. The baby, based on ultrasound, seems to be okay. She remains in the coma for two or three days, each day becoming more responsive. Does this make sense? Would there be long-term side effects? Are there any other tests or treatments they might perform?

A: Your scenario is not only possible but also likely.

What happens long term depends on the severity of the original trauma, the effectiveness of her treatment, and luck. She could have nothing more than a concussion, or she could have an intracranial bleed (bleeding within or around the brain) such as a subdural hematoma (the collection of blood between the brain and the

skull), which requires surgery. She could suffer severe and irreversible brain damage from lack of oxygen during the period that
she wasn't breathing, or she could recover with no long-term
impairment. From your description a simple concussion fits best.
People with concussions may wake up almost immediately or
remain in a coma for days, as in your situation.

Most likely she would recover well with only residual problems
such as headaches, some loss of cognitive function (thinking and
problem solving), and some difficulties with memory. These would
probably be minor and improve in a month or so. She likely would
not have any motor or sensory problems; that is, her legs, arms, and
other parts would work okay. She could develop a seizure disorder
from a brain scar left by the force of the trauma, but this would be
unlikely.

In the hospital an X ray of the skull and an MRI or CT brain
scan (with shielding of the abdomen by a lead apron to protect the
fetus from X-ray injury) would be done, and possibly a spinal tap
and an EEG (electroencephalogram—a test of brain wave activity).

She would be treated with IV medications such as steroids
(Solu-Medrol and Decadron are good ones) and possibly diuretics
(Lasix or Mannitol, most likely) to reduce any brain swelling, and
she would be watched for complications. That is about the only
treatment available or necessary.

The baby would be watched closely, and if any problems or signs
of fetal distress appeared, a cesarean section would be done. The
monitoring is accomplished by placing electrode patches, which
record the fetal heart rhythm and rate, on the mother's abdomen.
Also, a fetoscope would be fixed to the lower abdomen. This is an
ultrasound probe that images the fetus in real time using sound
waves and displays a picture of the baby on a small TV screen.
Signs of fetal distress would include an abnormal increase or
decrease or irregularity in the heart rate or rhythm and any abnormal movements by the fetus.

After recovery from the event, she may have some emotional

difficulties such as crying, irritability, anxiety attacks, and so forth. She may have insomnia, depression, and fits of anger. After all, she's still pregnant and worried about the health of the baby. She might blame herself for allowing this to happen or blame her husband for not being there—whatever fits the story.

Could Death from Bleeding Be Delayed for Several Days?

Q: My story takes place in a wagon train in the late 1800s. My character is dragged by a horse while crossing a river. He hits rocks and is bounced off the back wheel of a wagon. Of course the horse's hooves do damage as well. Three days later he dies due to massive bleeding from his internal injuries. This three-day delay followed by the sudden and dramatic loss of blood is important to the story's timing, but is it realistic?

A: The answer to your question is yes.

This type of accident could result in all types of injuries: broken bones, skull fractures, neck fractures, cracked ribs, punctured lungs, and intraabdominal injuries (injuries inside the abdominal cavity). This last type of injury might serve you well.

A ruptured spleen or lacerated liver or fractured kidney would bleed into the abdominal cavity. Death could be quick or take days if the bleed was slow. There would be great pain, especially with movement or breathing, and the abdomen would swell. Also a bluish bruiselike discoloration could appear around the umbilicus (belly button) and along the flanks. This usually takes twenty-four to forty-eight hours or more to appear and occurs as the blood seeps between the "fascial planes." The fascia are the tough white tissues that separate muscles from one another. The blood seeps along these divisions and reaches the deeper layers of the skin, causing the discoloration.

The problem for your scenario is that none of these types of internal injuries would lead to external bleeding. The abdominal cavity is a closed space, so the blood has no exit route.

However, if the injury was to the bowel, then external bleeding could occur. For blood to pass from the bowel, the bleeding would have to be within the bowel itself and not just in the abdomen somewhere. If the bowel was ruptured or torn so that bleeding occurred within the bowel, the blood would flow out rectally. But blood in the bowel acts like a laxative, so the bleeding would likely occur almost immediately and continue off and on until death, which in this situation would be minutes, hours, or a day, two at the most. It would be less realistic for the bleeding to wait three days before appearing in this case.

There is one exception, however, that may fit your story needs. The bowel could be bruised and not ruptured or torn, and a hematoma (blood mass or clot) could form in the bowel wall. As the hematoma expanded, it could compromise the blood supply to that section of the bowel. Over a day or two the bowel segment might die. We call this an "ischemic bowel." Ischemia is a term that means interruption of blood flow to an organ. If the bowel segment dies, bleeding would follow. This could allow a three-day delay in the appearance of blood.

In your scenario the injuries would likely be multiple, and so abdominal swelling, the discolorations I described, great pain, fevers, chills, delirium toward the end, and finally bleeding could all occur. This is not a pleasant way to die, but I imagine this happened not infrequently in frontier days.

The victim would be placed in the bed of one of the wagons and comforted as much as possible. He might be sponged with water to ease his fevers and offered water or soup, which he would likely vomit; prayers might also be said. He might be given tincture of opium (a liquid). This narcotic would also slow the motility (movement) of the bowel and thus lessen the pain and maybe the bleeding.

Of course, during the time period of your story, your characters wouldn't know any of the internal workings of the injury as I have described. They would only know that he was severely injured and in danger of dying. Some members of the wagon train might have seen similar injuries in the past and would know just how serious the victim's condition was, but they wouldn't understand the physiology behind it. They might even believe that after he survived the first two days he was going to live and then be very shocked when he eventually bled to death. Or they might understand that the bouncing of the wagon over the rough terrain was not only painful but also dangerous for someone in his condition. The train could be halted for the three days he lived, or several wagons could stay behind to tend to him while the rest of the column moved on.

What Was the Technique for Limb Amputation in the Nineteenth Century?

Q: My story takes place in the American frontier in the late 1800s. Near the end of the novel my protagonist must perform an amputation of an arm (a close-range gunshot wound at the elbow, with amputation just above the elbow). Can you tell me the typical procedure followed in an amputation? Blood vessels were badly damaged by the bullet, so I thought the protagonist would first apply a tourniquet. Is that okay? I'm letting the patient have a whiff of ether, so the surgeon may not have to rush through the job.

A: Amputations during the nineteenth century were dangerous and brutal. The ability to repair injured extremities and to control infections in gangrenous limbs did not exist at that time, and amputation was viewed as the only hope to save the victim. However, blood loss followed by shock and death or infection of the remaining stump dogged the surgeon's every effort. There was no blood to replace losses and treat shock, and antibiotics did not exist. Even with a successful procedure, the victim could die, and often did, from continued bleeding or infection.

The surgeon attempted to perform the procedure as rapidly as possible since it was very painful, and in frontier areas or during times of war anesthetic agents weren't readily available. A typical anesthetic was alcohol and sometimes tincture of opium or ether. Dr. Crawford Long first employed ether in surgery in Atlanta, Georgia, in 1842. The first public demonstration of its use took place in Boston in 1846, so it would be realistic for your protagonist to have access to it.

Even with a whiff of ether, the patient would likely have to be restrained by some of the stronger members of the community. A strip of leather or a piece of wood to bite down on might be employed.

As a medical student I scrubbed in on a couple of amputations. I came away with the impression that it remains a fairly brutal procedure with knives and saws and chisels and hammers. Yet even after those experiences, the most vivid image I have of this procedure is still the dramatic scene in *Gone with the Wind*.

Yes, a tourniquet would be tied very tightly around the extremity to prevent bleeding from the arteries that the surgeon would have to cut through. In your situation this would be done at the mid-humeral (upper arm) area. A large knife would be used to cut the tissues circumferentially (all the way around) down to the bone, and then a handsaw would complete the process. The stump would then be cauterized with a hot blade or other piece of metal heated over a fire and dressed with the cleanest pieces of cloth available.

The mortality rate for these procedures in the late 1800s was 50 percent or more. Most deaths occurred fairly quickly due to bleeding and shock; other victims lingered for days or weeks before succumbing to infection.

What Are the Physical Limitations of Someone with a Shoulder Dislocation?

Q: A character in a story I'm writing needs to be stuck in a remote hunting camp for two or three days with a dislocated shoulder. These are my questions:

1. If he doesn't get immediate treatment, will the damage continue to increase, or does the condition stay about the same?

2. What symptoms would he have? Will the immediate pain of the dislocation subside or get worse over the two to three days it goes untreated?

3. What kind of dysfunction will he have? Will he be able to use the arm at all? If he can't use or move the shoulder, will he still be able to grip things with the hand or lift very light objects?

4. When he does finally get treatment, exactly what is done for such an injury? How long will he be out of commission? If he was really tough, could he get back into action within a day or two?

A: The shoulder is one of the most—if not the most—complex joints in the body. Its range of motion is wide. It can hinge like the knee, rotate like the hip, and even whirl around in a circle like a windmill. It is basically a ball-and-socket joint, with the ball being the head of the humerus (upper arm bone) and the socket being formed by the glenoid cavity and the acromion of the scapula (shoulder blade). The above-mentioned portions of the scapula, the several ligaments that hold the humerus and the scapula together, and an inner lining of cartilage, which provides a smooth friction-free cuplike enclosure for the "ball" of the humerus to move within, form the joint capsule.

A dislocation occurs when the ball is forced out of the socket. Direct trauma to the shoulder or a severe torquing of the arm are the usual causes. Football players, gymnasts, and children yanked up by their arms are common victims of this type of shoulder injury.

The pain is immediate and severe, but once the dislocation has been "reduced" (the ball returned to the socket), the pain is minimal at that time. However, over the next several hours bleeding into the joint occurs, the muscles around the joint spasm (contract) in an attempt to stabilize the joint, and the pain returns. Any movement in any direction results in a knifelike stabbing pain in the shoulder. The first three or four days are the worst, but pain and limited motion may last for weeks or months. I have personal knowledge here—nine times. Football is a great sport.

Reducing the dislocation (manipulating or popping it back into place) can be accomplished in several ways. Sometimes merely raising the arm outward will pop it back into place. If another person is present, that person can drape the injured arm over his own shoulder (with the victim standing behind him) and lift the victim up on his back by bending forward. This pulls the humerus forward and outward, and often it will slip back into the socket. This can also be accomplished by laying the victim on his back, grasping his wrist, placing a foot against his chest near his axilla (armpit), and pulling his arm out to the side. This will pull the humeral head outward, and it often reseats itself in the socket. (Don't try any of these unless you know what you're doing because if it is done improperly, further injury may occur.) In your situation the victim could tie a rope around his wrist, attach the other end to a tree or rock, and pull the arm out to reduce the dislocation.

The sooner the shoulder dislocation is reduced, the better. Once the muscles spasm, reduction may be very difficult. Also, the nerves and blood vessels that go out to the arm pass beneath the shoulder, through the axilla. The pulse of the subclavian artery can be felt in the armpit. The dislocation can damage these vital conduits, and short- and long-term problems can result. Vascular damage can lead to ischemia (poor blood supply) of the arm, hematoma (a large collection of blood) formation, and possibly the development of an aneurysm (swelling of the artery). Nerve damage can cause loss of motor function (paralysis or weakness) and abnormal sensory function (numbness, tingling, loss of coordination, or diminished sense of touch and feel).

If the shoulder cannot be reduced, the injured person's limitations would be severe. He could not move the shoulder, and if the nerves were damaged or stretched, he might not be able to use his hand. If the dislocation was reduced, he would be able to function well for a few hours until the spasm sets in. After that the shoulder would be "frozen" and very painful with even the slightest movement. He should be able to bend his elbow and use his hands without a problem.

The typical treatment of a simple dislocation is to reduce it, place the arm in a sling, which is strapped to the chest to prevent shoulder movement, administer pain medications, and give it time to heal. If the injury is more complex, with severe damage to the joint capsule or with vascular or nerve injury, surgery may be required.

It would take several months for the shoulder to heal completely, but with a simple dislocation he should be able to move the shoulder carefully and do most things after a couple of weeks.

What Are the Symptoms and Treatment of a "Sucking Chest Wound"?

Q: I have a question about sucking chest wounds. I've written a scene in which a Vietnam War veteran applies a modified field dressing to his buddy's chest wound roughly ten minutes after the injury is sustained, but I

wonder if I'm stretching credibility by having my victim able to conduct a conversation with my hero. What
do you think? Is the injured man likely to survive?

A: First, let's look at "sucking chest wounds." I know, I know,
having any wound to the chest sucks, but there is a real medical
entity that goes by this moniker. Any object that penetrates the
chest wall and leaves behind an open wound would result in a
sucking chest wound. In a gunshot wound (GSW) to the chest, the
bullet typically makes a small hole as it travels through the tissues
of the chest wall. These tissues are elastic and tend to recoil and
collapse around the path of the bullet, closing it off and obliterat-
ing any opening to the outside. This may penetrate and collapse
the lung, and it may be fatal, but it isn't likely to produce a sucking
chest wound. The exit wound, however, may be large enough.

A larger wound, such as from explosive shrapnel or a spear or a
highway guardrail in an automobile accident or the above-
mentioned GSW exit wound, will not close in this fashion simply
due to the larger diameter of the wound. This leaves an opening to
the outside.

Breathing, drawing air into the lungs, depends on the production
of a negative pressure within the chest as the diaphragm lowers and
the chest expands. This pulls air into the lungs. During exhalation
this process is reversed, and air is forced back out of the lungs.
Close your mouth, pinch your nose, and try to breathe in and out.
Negative pressure during attempted inhalation and positive pressure during attempted exhalation are produced, but no air moves
because you have created a closed system and there is no opening
to the outside through which air can enter and exit.

With a wound that produces a large enough opening in the
chest wall, the normal expansion of the chest during inhalation
sucks air from the outside, through the wound, and into the chest
cavity, in the space between the lung and the chest wall. With
exhalation air is forced back through the opening and out of the

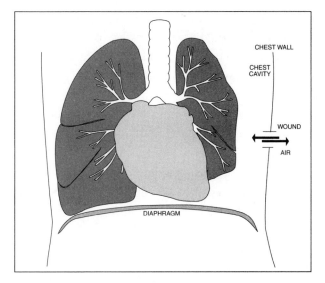

FIGURE 5. A SUCKING CHEST WOUND
Any injury that produces a large breach in the chest wall can result in
a "sucking chest wound." The positive and negative pressures created
within the chest cavity during breathing move air back and forth
through the wound, producing a "sucking" sound.

chest cavity (Figure 5). The lung on the injured side will collapse,
and a sucking sound is made with each inhalation and exhalation as
air moves back and forth through the wound—thus the name
"sucking chest wound." Fortunately, each lung is self-contained on
its side of the chest, so that the lung on the uninjured side will
remain inflated and function normally.

No, waiting ten minutes for help isn't a problem. Even an hour
is okay if the person is otherwise healthy. The victim would survive and be able to speak with only one lung for quite some time.
He would be short of breath, cough a lot, and be in pain, and fear
would be a big factor, but he would live.

The dressing applied should be "occlusive"; that is, it should seal
the opening in an airtight fashion. A porous gauze wouldn't do.
There are several types of plastic-coated bandages that stick to the
skin and make an airtight seal. Also, a sheet of plastic wrap, a plastic

food or trash bag, or a piece of cellophane would work. If only gauze is available, it should have some salve such as petroleum jelly, butter, or mud applied to it; that would make it airtight or nearly so.

If the lung itself wasn't also punctured, some re-expansion of the lung would occur while the victim awaited transport to a facility for definitive treatment. Once at the hospital a surgeon would repair the wound and place a thoracostomy tube (or chest tube). This large-bore plastic tube is slipped through the chest wall and into the chest cavity between the lung and the chest wall. Suction is applied to the tube in order to reinflate the lung. After a few days the tube is removed. The victim should recover and do well if this is his only injury.

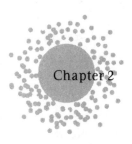

Chapter 2

ENVIRONMENTAL INJURIES AND THEIR TREATMENT

What Happens When Someone Dies from Exposure?

Q: What does it mean when someone dies of exposure—not freezing to death, just exposure?

A: "Exposure" is a broad term that covers deaths from freezing, heatstroke, starvation, and dehydration. In short, if the victim is in the middle of nowhere and doesn't die from injury or illness, then exposure is what did it. He didn't have food, water, or shelter. So to answer your specific question, if cold or heat isn't a factor, then lack of food and water is the likely culprit.

What Happens When Someone Dies from Dehydration?

Q: What's it like to die of dehydration? Delirium? Extreme thirst or the opposite? Does the mind fool the victim into seeing mirages? How long would this process take in an elderly woman lost in the mountains during the summer?

A: Dehydration is when the body loses water. This loss occurs due to sweating and through the lungs during normal breathing (called "insensible loss," since we are unaware of water lost in this fashion). The drier the air is and the more rapid the breathing, the more water will be lost through the lungs. Literally quarts of water can be lost this way. Any activity such as walking, running, carrying a backpack, or climbing increases the rate of breathing and, thus, insensible water loss. Hot and dry climates lead to more rapid water loss, though the dry air in winter mountains can cause considerable dehydration even though the temperature is low.

The time required for dehydration to appear depends on these and other factors. The process can take only hours if the weather is very hot and dry, or it can take a few days if it is cloudy and cooler.

In severe dehydration the blood pressure falls as the loss of water from the body reduces the blood volume. Also, electrolytes such as sodium, potassium, and magnesium are lost through sweating, which can lead to muscle weakness and cramps.

Thirst, an early symptom, doesn't appear until considerable loss of water has occurred. This means that by the time thirst develops, the person is already well into dehydration. Thirst is followed by fatigue, shortness of breath, weakness, muscle cramps, nausea and sometimes vomiting, delusions, delirium, and finally collapse, coma, and death.

With a high ambient temperature, body temperature can rise dramatically, and once it gets above 103 or so, the mind isn't as sharp as it should be. The victim will not be able to think well and may literally wander in circles or hallucinate. Mirages can be seen as a result.

Of course, mirages are due to the physics of light. Heat rising from a desert or a road bends light rays due to changes in density of the air (hot air is less dense than cooler air). The result is that you see blue sky below the horizon, and it looks like a body of water. Often a person who is dehydrated and confused will rush blindly toward it but can never reach it because it doesn't exist and because the optical illusion keeps moving away, so to speak.

The young and the old are particularly susceptible to dehydration and heatstroke since they tend to have less muscle and tissue mass in which to store water. They dehydrate faster and show the signs and symptoms of dehydration earlier and more severely.

In your scenario both the summer heat and the altitude would conspire to hasten your lady's dehydration. The heat would increase sweating, and the low water vapor pressure (meaning the air is dry) that is found at higher altitudes would accelerate insensible loss of water through the lungs. Another factor would be her degree of hydration at the time her adventure began. If she was already a little dry, she would get into trouble more quickly. Also, as explained above, the more active she is, the faster she would dehydrate. If she sits in a cool spot and waits for someone to find her, she might survive for several days. If she attempts to walk over hilly terrain, she might not last twenty-four hours. Obviously, if she has any underlying heart or lung disease or perhaps diabetes, her survival time would decrease.

What Is the Treatment for Dehydration?

Q: What's the first aid treatment for dehydration? In my story a forest ranger comes across a severely dehydrated and weakened hiker. He carries the young man to safety. But what would he actually do? Dribble water between his lips and get him to a hospital? Then what? An IV with a glucose drip?

A: That's right. Get water in any way you can safely do it, such as sips or dribbles at first, depending on the condition and level of consciousness of the victim. Other treatment depends on whether heat prostration or heatstroke is present.

If the environment is cool or cold, as in the mountains or snowy areas, wrap the victim in blankets, towels, or sweaters since dehydration in these circumstances often leads to a drop in body temperature. Typically, the victim of this type of dehydration feels cool to the touch and appears pale. If the dehydration is severe, the blood pressure will be low and the pulse weak and thready, and confusion and disorientation are likely. Giving fluids (preferably warm liquids) and warming the victim are the major frontline treatments.

In your story, heat prostration and heatstroke are more likely since the ambient temperature is high. These two entities are similar, with the latter being more severe. Both are caused by dehydration and rising core body temperature. Common victims include runners, football players, construction workers, military personnel, and anyone who exerts himself in hot climates, such as your hiker. Sweating in these situations is typically profuse, so dehydration can occur rapidly.

We use the term "heat injury" as a broad category for anyone who develops significant dehydration and an elevation of body temperature. Early in heat injury (heat prostration) the victim may sweat, but as the process continues and the core body temperature rises, sweating ceases, compounding the problem by the loss of the body's natural radiator system (resulting in heatstroke). The reason this occurs is that the body's innate self-preservation actions divert what blood volume there is toward vital organs such as the heart and brain, and away from the skin. But it is blood flow through the skin that acts as the radiator to dissipate the rising body heat. The body actually works against itself, and the core temperature rises rapidly. Body temperatures of 105 to 108 are not uncommon. Thus, victims of heatstroke may appear flushed and often feel warm and dry to the touch. Heatstroke has a high mortality if not treated quickly and aggressively.

Whether the victim is suffering from heat prostration or heatstroke, the treatment is directed toward lowering the body temperature and replacing the lost fluids. These measures should begin immediately and should not be delayed in order to transport the victim to a hospital. Cool the victim by sponging with water or any cool liquid, and fan with a towel, shirt, or anything handy. This lowering of the core body temperature is as important as relieving the dehydration by giving fluids. In fact, when a victim of heatstroke appears in the hospital emergency room, we often place him in a tub of ice water to rapidly lower the core body temperature. The brain does not tolerate the high temperatures seen in heatstroke, and irreversible brain damage occurs quickly.

A victim who is in a coma or delirious or confused and combative is another problem. Pouring water into the mouth of a comatose person or one who will not cooperate may lead to aspiration and injury to the lungs. It's a judgment call as to which is the greater risk: untreated dehydration or aspiration.

Your forest ranger would likely have a canteen or some other water container. He would give the victim sips, splash some on his face and chest, and fan him with a shirt or similar object. He would move him into the shade of nearby trees and then transport him to civilization by whatever means he had available. He might call in a helicopter rescue team or make a litter and haul the victim down the mountain. Regardless, he would continue to rehydrate and cool the hiker as long as his water supply lasted.

In the hospital the victim would receive IV fluids, usually D5W, which is 5 percent dextrose in water, or D5½ NS (normal saline,) which is 5 percent dextrose in salt water that has half the salt (NaCl) content of blood.

Other electrolytes such as potassium and magnesium can be added to the IV as needed, depending on the results of blood tests for these minerals. Tests of kidney function are also important since dehydration and heat injury can damage them.

How Long Can Someone Survive in a Freezer?

Q: Say I want to shove a character in a commercial freezer. How long would it take for the poor soul to die?

A: The time required depends on so many factors that no definitive answer is possible. Here are some factors that would impact survival:

Size and weight of the victim: This is a situation where a high percent of body fat would be welcome. Fat serves as insulation and a source of energy for heat production by the body.

Age: The very young and the very old would tolerate the cold poorly and be at greater risk.

Diseases the victim may have: The presence of heart or vascular disease, diabetes, or anemia would likely hasten the victim's demise.

Food and beverage intake: When and what was the last meal? A high-carbohydrate meal might help somewhat. If the victim was well hydrated, he would be better off than if he was dehydrated. Alcohol consumption would definitely hasten loss of body heat and quicken the demise

Medications or drugs: Alcohol, as mentioned, and some other medications can hasten heat loss from the body. Diuretics lead to dehydration, and certain blood pressure medications dilate the body's blood vessels and thus increase heat loss.

Clothing: A ski parka would be better than a cotton Hawaiian shirt.

Temperature within the freezer: Pray it's defective. If it is simply a cold locker for vegetable storage, the ambient temperature would be above freezing. If it was a meat or frozen food freezer, the temperature would be well below freezing and maybe below 0 degrees. A circulating fan in the freezer would definitely shorten the survival time. Think windchill.

Protective materials present: Any cloth, canvas, or covering inside the freezer that could be used as a coat or to build an "ice cave" would be helpful. Either would help retain body heat.

Perhaps you can use some of these to make the victim's survival longer or shorter as dictated by your story requirements. In general, two hours probably wouldn't be enough, and forty-eight would be plenty. I suggest leaving the victim in overnight if he is an average person and not dressed for the Antarctic. That'd probably do it.

Many people survive for days lost in blizzards or in the mountains during the winter. Others don't make it through the first twelve hours. Your victim could do either, depending on what you want.

Does Alcohol Intake Prevent Death from Freezing?

Q: Does this make sense medically? A man falls through the ice of a frozen lake at night. He is unable to get himself out but has a bottle of brandy in his pocket, which he sips through the night and survives until he is rescued the next morning. Would the alcohol help him survive? Would it act like antifreeze?

A: Sorry, but your character is doomed, and his actions would only hasten his demise. Let me explain.

Our skin serves as our radiator. In hot weather the capillaries in the skin dilate, blood flow through the skin increases, and heat is lost to the atmosphere. That is why many people look flushed when they are warm. The evaporation of sweat consumes some of the heat since turning a liquid into a gas (evaporation) requires energy, and it is the body heat that supplies this energy. Thus, heat is lost. People suffering from heat prostration or heatstroke are bathed with water and fanned with a towel or whatever is available.

This promotes evaporation and heat loss from the overheated body of the victim.

Cold is the exact opposite. The body attempts to hold its heat. Blood is diverted away from the skin so that less heat is lost through "the radiator." That is why people look paler when they are cold. When exposed to extremes of cold, the best way to protect yourself from freezing is to cover up, stay out of the wind (moving air absorbs more of the heat), and create warmer ambient air by building an ice cave or burrow of some kind. This traps the body's heat in the "cocoon," and thus less is lost. In water this isn't possible. Similar to a cold wind, the movement of the water or the victim's movements within the water would greatly increase heat loss. During World War II the survival of pilots shot down in the North Atlantic could be measured in minutes.

Now to the brandy issue.

Alcohol dilates the vessels in the skin, which increases blood flow and thus heat loss. Some people become flushed after alcohol consumption. This seems to be especially true with red wine, but it happens with any alcohol. In a cold environment this is the exact opposite of what is desired. The old image of the Saint Bernard with a cask of brandy hanging from his neck is bad medicine. Alcohol hastens heat loss, and thus death from freezing.

Alcohol does not act as antifreeze in the human bloodstream.

In your scenario the man would be up to his neck in frigid water and would likely thrash around in an attempt to stay afloat. The icy water would rapidly dissipate his body heat, and he would become hypothermic (low body temperature) in a matter of ten to twenty minutes, maybe less. If he drank the brandy or was intoxicated before he took the plunge, this time would be shortened considerably. Symptoms of hypothermia include fatigue, weakness, lethargy, and confusion. His strength and coordination would diminish and his survival struggles weaken, and he would drown.

You may remember the dramatic news video of the young woman being rescued from an icy Potomac River. When she was thrown a line, she was too weak to grip it and sank beneath the water. Fortunately, a heroic man jumped in and saved her. Unless your character had such a hero handy, he would succumb to the cold and drown.

Could your guy survive? Not likely, but there is an old Emergency Department adage that says, "You can't kill a drunk." That is why when you read about a drunk driver hitting a carload of people, it's always the family that dies, never the drunk. Sometimes life doesn't make sense.

Could Someone Survive in a Roadway Tunnel Where a Forest Fire Raged at Both Ends?

Q: This is going to sound like an odd question, but what would happen to a character trapped in a roadway tunnel that cuts through a hillside while a forest fire raged on either end? Would he survive? Would he get burned?

A: Survival would depend on the length and size of the tunnel, whether the fire raged at both ends, whether there was a vent that was away from the fire so that fresh air could be obtained, and other factors. The two dangers would be cooking from the heat and suffocation from the fire consuming the oxygen. If your victim had underlying heart or lung disease, his survival time would be shortened.

The bigger the tunnel, the more air he would have and the farther away from the fire he could stay. If the fire blazed at both ends of the tunnel, it would rapidly consume all the oxygen from the air in the tunnel, and he would suffocate unless a source of fresh air was available—either natural or via some form of breathing apparatus. If it burned only at one end or if a vent was present that was away from the flames, these sources of fresh air would increase his chance of survival. Also, this situation might give him an escape route.

In a short tunnel surrounded by fire, the victim would likely suffocate and cook.

Forest fire fighters carry protective blankets to crawl under and bottled air to breathe just in case the fire overruns them. In most cases this gives them enough protection to survive long enough for the fire to move on. The same could be true for your character. If the tunnel insulated him from the heat and if a source of fresh air was available, he might survive long enough for the fire to move on. Otherwise, he wouldn't.

What Happens When Someone Is Struck by Lightning?

Q: In my story I have a character who is struck by lightning but survives. What kind of injuries might he suffer? What long-term problems would follow?

A: Lightning strikes come in four varieties.

1. *Direct strike*: The lightning hits the victim directly. This is the most serious type and is more likely if the victim is holding a metal object such as a golf club or umbrella.

2. *Flashover*: The lightning travels over the outside of the body. This is more likely if the victim is wearing wet clothing or is covered with sweat.

3. *Side flash:* The current "splashes" from a nearby building, tree, or other person and then spreads to the victim.

4. *Stride potential:* The lightning strikes the ground near the victim, who has one foot closer to the strike than the other. This sets up a potential electrical difference between the legs called a "stride potential." The current enters through one leg, spreads through the body, and exits via the other leg.

When dealing with lightning, which is a direct current, the numbers involved are huge. The voltage varies from 3 million to 200 million volts, and the amperes range from 2,000 to 3,000. Quite a jolt. Fortunately, the current is very brief, averaging from 1 to 100 milliseconds (thousandths of a second).

The injuries that result are primarily due to the massive electrical current and the body's conversion of the electrical energy to heat. The electrical shock can literally stop the heart or cause dangerous and deadly changes in heart rhythm. The heat can burn and char the skin, scorch the clothing, and fuse or melt metal objects in the victim's pockets, buttons on his shirt, belt buckles, and fillings in his teeth.

All the tissues of the body are susceptible to injury. The skin may be charred and even display entry and exit burns. The heart muscle may be damaged and scarred. The liver, kidneys, bone marrow, and muscles may suffer permanent injuries. The brain and spinal cord may be damaged, and residual weakness in an arm or leg is not uncommon. Loss of memory and psychiatric difficulties may follow.

One interesting sign of lightning strikes that rarely occurs are Lichtenberg Figures (Figure 6), which were first described by German physicist Georg Christoph Lichtenberg in 1777. This is a painless red fernlike or arboresque pattern over the back, shoulders, buttocks, or legs. It tends to fade over a couple of days, leaving behind no scars or discolorations. It is uncommon but fascinating.

Treatment depends on the severity of the injuries. The first order of business is to reestablish breathing and heart rhythm if either or both are absent. Steroids are given to lessen swelling and inflammation in the body's organs. Burns are treated in the usual fashion with cleaning and dressing as indicated. Blood tests would assess the degree of liver, kidney, and muscle damage. When muscles are injured in this fashion, the muscle cells may die or rupture. If so, they release their internal myoglobin and other proteins into the bloodstream. These proteins can severely damage the kidneys because the kidneys attempt to filter them from the blood. Flush-

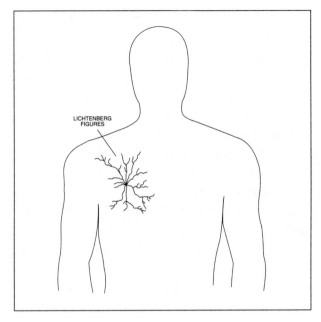

FIGURE 6. LICHTENBERG FIGURES
Lichtenberg Figures are a rare consequence of lightning injury. They are painless red fernlike patterns on the skin that tend to fade over a few days and leave no permanent markings.

ing the kidneys with a large amount of IV fluids may prevent kidney failure.

Recovery can be complete, with no residual problems, or the victim may have permanent liver, kidney, cardiac, psychiatric, or neurologic problems. Luck and rapid, effective treatment are important here.

Can a Person Stranded at Sea Survive by Drinking His Own Urine?

Q: If someone was stranded in the desert or on a life raft in the open sea, could he survive by drinking his own urine. Is it dangerous or toxic? Or is it okay?

A: Any port in a storm, so to speak.

Yes, this would help—at first. Urine is simply water with impurities that have been filtered from the blood by the kidneys. In the type of exposure you describe, dehydration is the major problem. Any source of water would be beneficial. However, the concentration of impurities in the urine would increase as dehydration progressed, and very quickly the urine would supply more toxins than water. Drinking it would then be counterproductive.

In reality by the time a person considered drinking his own urine, he would already be severely dehydrated, his urine would be very concentrated, and consuming it would be of little benefit.

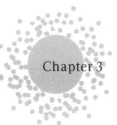

Chapter 3

DOCTORS, HOSPITALS, AND
PARAMEDICAL PERSONNEL

Can X-Ray Films Be Copied?

Q: Can an X ray be photocopied or otherwise duplicated?

A: Yes. X rays are often copied by use of a special copier designed for this purpose. Most hospital radiology departments have such capability, and it takes only a few minutes. Also, nowadays many hospitals acquire and store the images in a digital format. These can be duplicated, printed, altered, e-mailed, and all the other things one can do with digital data.

How Do Doctors Handle Emergencies and Concussions?

Q: In an emergent medical situation, what initial questions might a doctor ask? And if he suspects the person might have sustained a concussion or a more serious head injury, what specific questions might he ask?

A: The initial questions are similar regardless of what the emergent situation is. The key is to get as much information as possible in the shortest time and with the fewest questions. In true emergencies time is often the enemy, and the physician doesn't have the luxury of taking a long history from the patient. I always taught my students that in such situations you can get most of the information you absolutely need with the following three questions:

1. *What's wrong or what happened?* We call this the "chief complaint." Seventy percent of the time the diagnosis can be narrowed to a very few choices with the answer to this question. A complaint of chest pain leads you in one direction or line of thinking, nausea in another, and headache in yet another.

2. *Have you ever been hospitalized or treated for anything in the past, and if so, for what?* We call this the "past medical history." The answer tells the M.D. about the medical problems that the person has experienced in the past and gives him the necessary background to evaluate the current problem. Many of the patient's past illnesses will have an effect on his current illness or injury, and, indeed, many of these past illnesses may still be active medical problems. Heart disease and diabetes would fall into this category since they don't go away but, rather, tend to progress.

3. *Do you take any medications or have any allergies?* This tells the M.D. what the active medical problems are, such as high blood pressure, diabetes, heart disease, hepatitis, and so forth, and how they are being treated or managed. This information also guides the M.D.'s treatment so he can avoid drug interactions and the use of known allergic drugs.

These are the general questions a physician asks of any patient in an emergency situation. If the victim is not conscious, much of this information can be obtained from relatives, friends, another M.D. who knows the patient, or medical records. MedicAlert bracelets are also helpful.

After this basic data is obtained, more pointed questions are asked to fill in the areas of concern. For a patient with a head injury, the following questions are essential:

> Do you have a headache? Is it localized or general?
> Do you have blurred or abnormal vision?
> Are you experiencing dizziness or poor balance?
> Have you been nauseous or vomiting?
> Do you have any soreness or stiffness in the neck?
> Do you feel any weakness? Is it generalized or only in one side, arm, or leg?
> Are your eyes sensitive to light?
> Do any of these symptoms worsen with a change in position or movement?

Then, of course, a complete physical and neurologic exam is performed. Based on the answers and the findings on the exam, lab work, X rays, and other tests would be obtained as indicated.

How Do Hospitals Ration the Blood Supply in Major Natural Disasters?

Q: I have an odd question for you. Let's say the big one hit Los Angeles tomorrow, devastating the city. I imagine the blood supply would be depleted rather quickly. How aggressive would doctors be about getting blood donors? Would doctors at temporary M.A.S.H.-like medical facilities solicit healthy people off the street to give blood? Would they be able to screen this blood quickly for AIDS?

A: Every hospital has an emergency or disaster plan that deals with catastrophes such as an earthquake. That said, whenever a major event such as you describe occurs, these plans may be over-taxed and become quickly inadequate.

M.A.S.H.-like field hospitals would crop up out of necessity, and the blood supply would be rapidly consumed. The Red Cross and other organizations would transport blood, and volunteer donors would be called in. The Red Cross keeps a list of clean donors that they regularly call on when needed; blood would be obtained from them. Yes, people off the street might be used. So far, so good. Labs would be set up to supplement those of the local hospitals to type and match the blood and screen it for AIDS and hepatitis.

Screening for hepatitis and AIDS cannot be done quickly. Several hours and up to a day or two would be required. As the injured rolled in, it would be necessary for these considerations to take a backseat. After all, would you rather bleed to death or risk the very small possibility of contracting hepatitis or AIDS?

At some point all this would not be enough, and unmatched (type specific) and untested blood would have to be used to save some lives. Type-specific blood is the same type that the patient has, but it does not have full cross-matching of all possible incompatibil-ities. It takes only a few minutes and very little equipment to deter-mine if blood is O-negative, for example, but it is more involved to actually test the donor blood against that of the recipient for true compatibility. This increases the possibility of a reaction, but this sit-uation exemplifies the old adage: "Any port in a storm."

What Is Artificial Blood?

Q: While on a safari in Africa, one of my characters is attacked and severely injured by a crocodile. His leg is mauled, and he nearly bleeds to death before he is evac-uated to a hospital. I've read recently about artificial blood and may want to incorporate it in my story. What is artificial blood? Is it available? Are there any problems?

A: Artificial blood has been the subject of research for three decades. The concerns regarding AIDS and hepatitis, the erratic availability and difficulty in storing and transporting real blood, and the need for blood in remote areas such as war zones has driven this research.

First a word about what artificial blood is and isn't. It is a product that supplies molecules capable of carrying oxygen from the lungs to the tissues and bringing carbon dioxide back to the lungs to be expelled. The normal IV fluids given to patients in shock or those suffering from blood loss are basically water with some electrolytes (sodium, potassium, and so forth) and sugar, and they have no ability to carry oxygen, which is the immediate concern in shock situations. Artificial blood is designed to fill this need.

However, artificial blood is not real blood. It does not contain vitamins, nutrients, hormones, antibodies, platelets (small blood cells involved in clotting), or any of the proteins involved in the clotting of blood. If given injudiciously or in large amounts, it will dilute these needed clotting factors and lead to a worsening of the bleeding, which would be counterproductive. Artificial blood is used as a bridge to stabilize the victim long enough to get him to a proper medical facility, where definitive treatment can be rendered and real blood given.

Early attempts at developing artificial blood revolved around extracting the hemoglobin molecule and modifying it so that it could be given without giving the entire red blood cell (RBC), which must be stored and refrigerated. Hemoglobin is the molecule within the RBCs that binds, carries, and releases oxygen and carbon dioxide. Unfortunately, the hemoglobin molecule when removed from the RBCs is very toxic and causes an increase in mortality. A report in the November 17, 1999, issue of the *Journal of the American Medical Association* showed that such a product, called HemAssist (Baxter Healthcare), when used in trauma patients led to a mortality rate of 46 percent as compared to a rate of only 17 percent in those who received the typical IV fluids. It was back to the drawing board.

Several other products are under development and being tested at this time. One of the most promising is called Hemopure, which is produced by the Biopure Corporation in Cambridge, Massachusetts. It was recently approved for use in South Africa but as yet is not available in the United States. Hemopure is based on hemoglobin extracted from the RBCs of cow blood. Unlike whole blood, it doesn't need to be refrigerated and has a shelf life of two years (42 days is usual for properly refrigerated blood). Its administration is simple: Start an IV and drip it in.

In your story it would be perfectly reasonable for the medical personnel on your safari to have available Hemopure or any similar product your imagination might create. This is fiction, after all. As long as artificial blood has some factual basis, which it does, you can make up your own brand name.

Your crocodile victim would be removed from the croc's mouth; his wounds would be treated with local compression and tourniquets to control the bleeding; he would be given intravenous fluids (probably D5LR—5 percent dextrose in lactated Ringer's solution) and a couple of bottles of Hemopure (or Product XYZ); and transported to a hospital facility. There, he would receive real blood and undergo surgery to repair his injuries. The artificial blood would be the bridge that allows him to survive.

What Is Blood Doping, and How Does It Work?

Q: I'm writing a story in which a young track star uses the process of blood doping to gain an unfair advantage in an upcoming meet. How is blood doping done? Are there any complications?

A: Athletic performance and endurance are dependent on the ability of the body to supply oxygen and nutrients to working muscles and remove toxic by-products from them. This requires a conditioned cardiovascular system, an adequate supply of glycogen and other energy sources from the liver and muscles, and blood rich in hemoglobin, the molecule in red blood cells (RBCs) that carries the oxygen from the lungs to the muscles. The more hemoglobin in the blood, the better it transports oxygen.

The natural way to increase the RBCs and hemoglobin is to live or train at an altitude where the thinner air stimulates the bone marrow to produce more RBCs. People in Denver, Colorado, tend to have a greater concentration of RBCs and hemoglobin in their blood than those who live at sea level. An athlete who moves to the mountains to train would see results after a few weeks.

Blood doping is a method of doing this artificially. It is basically the removal of blood, separating and storing the RBCs, and giving the plasma back. After three or four weeks the body has replaced the removed RBCs. Then, at a later date, the stored RBCs are given. This immediately increases the concentration of RBCs (and hemoglobin) in the blood, which improves oxygen delivery capacity and thus athletic performance. Marathoners, cyclists, and other endurance athletes can use this procedure to gain an unfair advantage.

Complications are rare if the process is handled appropriately. Transfusion reactions do not occur since the person is receiving his own blood. However, if the blood is mishandled, problems can arise. If the blood is inadequately stored or if its sterility is violated, bacteria can grow in the stored blood and cause septicemia (infection in the bloodstream) when infused. This can lead to severe illness and death. If the blood is frozen or agitated, both of which can damage or shatter the RBCs, kidney damage can result when the blood is given.

Some athletes shortcut this process by taking a transfusion of someone else's blood. There is no removal of their own blood and no three-week wait to rebuild their own blood count. But this raises the problem of a transfusion reaction, which can happen even if the blood is adequately cross-matched. It was alleged that during the 1984 Olympics, some members of the U.S. cycling team blood-doped a week or so before their competition. They apparently didn't have time to do it properly and used type-specific blood donated by relatives and friends. This blood of the same type (for example, O-negative), which has not been matched for compatibility against the recipient's own blood, greatly increases the chance of a reaction, not to mention the transmission of hepatitis or AIDS.

Physicians use type-specific blood in only the direst of medical emergencies, situations where there just isn't time for a complete cross-match because the patient is bleeding to death. You do what's necessary in these circumstances and then deal with the consequences. A bicycle race hardly qualifies.

Another substance used for this type of performance enhancement is recombinant erythropoietin. Erythropoietin occurs naturally in the human body and stimulates the production of RBCs. It is manufactured by recombinant DNA techniques and, when injected, artificially increases the RBC count. Medically it is used in patients with chronic kidney failure where anemia is common and difficult to treat.

One problem that can arise in blood doping, regardless of the method, is a thickening of the blood. The more RBCs the blood contains, the more viscous it is. In fact, there are several medical conditions, such as polycythemia vera, where the concentration of RBCs becomes so great that the patient must be bled. We call this a phlebotomy. Yes, Renaissance medicine still lives. If the blood becomes too thick, it can literally sludge in the capillaries and cause strokes, heart attacks, kidney damage, and loss of digits. It can happen to an athlete whose exercise leads to dehydration if his blood is artificially thickened.

An athlete can botch the process and have a transfusion reaction, damage his kidneys, or become infected, or he can successfully complete the blood doping only to suffer a fatal heart attack during the competition. Or he can get away with it and win the race.

What Is the Basic Procedure for Blood Donation?

Q: It has been a few years since I donated blood. What is the basic medical procedure for drawing your blood? What questions do they ask beforehand?

A: Review the answer to the question regarding the basic medical questions a physician asks in emergent situations. These are important in the donor situation since certain current and past medical problems and the taking of some medications preclude the donation of blood. Other questions are designed to determine the presence or possible presence of any transmittable diseases such as hepatitis or AIDS.

The procedure is basic. A large-bore needle (14 or 16 gauge) is introduced into a vein in the soft depression on the inside of the elbow (called the antecubital fossa). The blood is then drawn into a bottle or plastic bag. The needle is removed and a bandage placed. The major concern for the donor is dizziness or fainting. Some people develop what is called the Vasovagal Syndrome. This is what happens when someone sees blood and faints. It is caused by a massive outpouring of stimuli from the brain, which excites the vagus nerve. This nerve exits the stem of the brain and wanders (like a "vagrant," thus the name) through the body, enervating the heart, lungs, blood vessels, and most of the gastrointestinal tract. It is involved with the regulation of blood pressure, heart rate, and a multitude of other bodily functions. When it is stimulated, the blood vessels dilate (open up), and the heart rate and blood pressure may drop dramatically, leading to dizziness and loss of consciousness.

Also, the removal of a pint of blood in a short period of time decreases the blood volume—the old "quart low" phenomenon. This can also lead to dizziness when the person stands. That is why orange juice or some other fluid is given and the donor is watched for a half hour or so. This gives the body time to rebalance the blood volume.

Over the next few weeks the body revs up the bone marrow to replace the donated blood, and life goes on. Donations should not be made any more often than every six weeks or so to prevent the development of iron deficiency and anemia in the donor.

What Medical Emergency That Required Quick Action Would Likely Occur in a Gunshot Victim in a Hospital ICU?

Q: I'm writing a scene in which a paramedic is contemplating pulling the plug on a critically ill bad guy in the hospital ICU. Just as he decides to do so, however, the bad guy (a gunshot victim, by the way) suffers some kind of life-threatening emergency (cardiac arrest?), and the paramedic, acting strictly on impulse, performs some form of medical heroics to save the guy's life before hospital staff can reach his room.

Can you suggest a viable set of circumstances to fit such a scenario? What type of life-threatening emergency would specifically fit the bill here, and what could our paramedic do to avert disaster in the fifteen or so seconds it is likely to take the staff to respond to the situation?

A: A cardiac arrest would be perfect. Sudden and intense, it can be remedied with a single quick response. The paramedic could be at the bedside, contemplating his actions, when the monitor above the bed shows a sudden change in the intended victim's cardiac

rhythm. It can be either ventricular tachycardia or ventricular fibrillation. An alarm would sound in the room and at the nurses' station. The nurse watching the monitors at the station would see the
same tracing, recognize the need for emergent intervention, and
immediately a Code Blue would be called over the hospital speaker
system: "Code Blue, ICU 3! Code Blue, ICU 3!"

The Code Blue team typically consists of ICU and/or ER
nurses, the ER physician or any M.D. on the floor, a respiratory
technician, and other ancillary personnel. They race to the room
with a "crash cart" that has all the medicines, IV fluids, portable
defibrillator, and so forth, needed for a resuscitation.

Meanwhile, the paramedic could act. A portable defibrillator
unit would likely be at the bedside. He could grab the paddles,
place them on the patient's chest, and fire away. The single shock
could immediately return the person's rhythm to normal so that
when the nurses and others arrived, the crisis would already be
over. The doctor would then examine the patient and request an
EKG, lab work, and other items in an effort to figure out why the
event occurred.

Another possibility would be to have another Code Blue going
on down the hall or in another ICU cubicle. Maybe when the victim's cardiac arrest occurs and the alarm goes off, a young and
inexperienced nurse or a nurse's aide can run into the room and say
the code team is tied up. He then can enlist her help (this would
give you an opportunity for some interaction or dialog if that
works for you), or he tells her to get one of the ICU nurses from
the other Code Blue. After she runs out of the room to get help, he
realizes he can't wait and must act now or the man will die.

This would be a likely real-life occurrence. I remember one wild
night as an intern when we had three codes on the same floor at
once. To say the resources were stretched thin would be an under-
statement.

What Information Would Emergency Department Personnel Give Out Regarding a "John Doe"?

Q: In my current novel my character's husband is missing. She calls the hospital, which informs her that there is a John Doe there matching his description. She immediately goes to the hospital to take a look.

My questions: Would they mention over the phone that they have a man fitting her husband's description? Is there a procedure for her to see and talk with this person, or would she just be allowed to take a look?

A: I assume that the man would be injured or unconscious or amnesiac or confused. Otherwise, he could tell them who he was and give permission to notify his wife. The police may be present in such a circumstance, especially if some sort of trauma is involved.

The charge nurse or the emergency room (ER) doctor would likely tell the caller that there was a John Doe in the ER but wouldn't give too many details—nothing that would violate patient confidentiality. But since the ER personnel and perhaps the police don't know who the person is and would be trying to identify him, anyone who could do so would be helpful. They would likely ask that she come to the ER.

When she arrives, the nurse or the doctor would probably let her see the victim. Remember, the doctor is responsible for the man's care, and he would want all the information he can get. Having a family member or friend identify the victim is a huge step in that direction. He could then ask about the victim's past medical history, allergies, current medical problems, current medications, and so forth—in other words, the things he needs to know to care for the patient.

What Medical Expertise Would a Seasoned Commando Possess?

Q: I have a character who served as a commando in the Israeli special forces and was specifically trained as a medic. He spent time in war zones where he carried out medical treatments for which he was not officially trained. His strategic skills quickly gave him an international reputation for planning and executing daring raids, rescues, and so on. While I rarely use his medical skills in the stories, I want to be accurate when I do. It seems he would be midway between someone with Boy Scout or Red Cross first aid skills and a medical doctor. Realistically, what would be the limits of this man's medical abilities?

A: His medical skills could be almost any level you wish. His abilities would be at least those of a well-trained paramedic. He would know CPR and how to handle many types of emergency situations. Since he served as a combat medic, he should be able to perform the initial treatment for all types of war injuries—wounds caused by gunshots, shrapnel, knives, explosives, and others. He would be adept at controlling bleeding, maintaining an airway, stabilizing fractures, and suturing most superficial lacerations. His biggest asset would be his grace under fire. When faced with any serious injury or emergent situation, the first step is to avoid panic and use common sense. That goes for M.D.s, too. He should be well equipped in this regard.

If you avoid the temptation of allowing him to perform sophisticated surgeries and treatments, you should be okay regardless of what he does.

Can Firefighters Estimate the Survival Time of a Victim Trapped in an Airtight Enclosure?

Q: An amateur illusionist walls himself up in a very small space in his basement, assuring his wife he can free himself without assistance. Naturally, she calls 911 so that rescue personnel can get him out. My question: How would firefighters arriving on the scene estimate how much oxygen he had left in the enclosed space? Is there a calculation they use based on the space in cubic feet, the height and weight of the trapped individual, and other information? If he was a diabetic and forgot to take his insulin with him, how would this complicate the situation?

A: Estimate? Maybe. Calculate? No way. This situation is much too complex. Let me explain.

First, the physiology. In the simplest of terms, the lungs take in air, transport oxygen (O_2) from this air into the bloodstream, remove carbon dioxide (CO_2) from the blood and exhale it back into the environment. This simple process is actually very complex and requires good air, good lungs, a good circulatory system, plenty of red blood cells, and a ton of chemical reactions. The diseases that can interfere with this process are numerous. In your scenario, however, we are dealing with a healthy person who has normal lungs and other criteria.

Unfortunately, that doesn't simplify the calculation very much. Let's take a glimpse at just how complicated such a calculation can be.

I'm sorry, but the metric system must be used here. Remember that one meter (m) is about 39 inches (3 feet 3 inches) and equals

100 centimeters (cm). A cubic centimeter (cc) is a measure of volume. One cc is a volume that is 1 cm × 1 cm × 1 cm.

Air at sea level is 21 percent oxygen.

An airtight room that is 3 m × 3 m × 3 m (roughly 9 feet on all sides) would contain 27 cubic meters (or 27,000,000 cc) of air and about 5.67 cubic meters (5,670,000 cc) of oxygen.

A normal breath is about 500 cc. However, about 30 percent of each breath never reaches the alveoli (air sacs) and thus isn't involved in gas exchange (the passage of oxygen from the lungs into the bloodstream). This is the air that fills the bronchi (breathing tubes), which is termed the "anatomic dead space." Thus, 70 percent of each breath is potentially useful. Since an individual at rest breathes approximately 16 times a minute at 500 cc per breath, these are the calculations:

$$\text{Total air intake } = 500 \times 16 = 8000 \text{ cc}$$
$$\text{"Useful" air intake } = 8000 \times 70\% = 5600 \text{ cc}$$
$$\text{Oxygen intake } = 5600 \times 21\% = 1176 \text{ cc}$$

A person at rest therefore inhales about 1176 cc of oxygen per minute. This means that the oxygen in the room would last about 4821 minutes, or 80 hours (5,760,000 divided by 1176).

It seems like a long time to survive in an airtight box, doesn't it? It is.

These calculations assume that the person could use every cc of oxygen in the room. Not so. Remember that with each breath the percent of the air that is oxygen drops, and the concentration of carbon dioxide rises. By the time the O_2 concentration fell to 15 percent or so, the person would be in severe trouble. This means that only about 6 percent (21 minus 15) of the oxygen content can be used to calculate survival time. And, of course, the mounting CO_2 level compounds the problem.

When you add to this the fact that bigger people have higher O_2

requirements and that any activity, even standing or walking, increases O_2 usage, the calculations become extremely complex. And we've considered only the basic physiologic components of this situation. There are many others that are simply too intricate to explain. So even though these calculations can be done, they are not easy and cannot be performed by firefighters trying to save someone.

As you can see, this is a nice exercise in math and physiology, but it doesn't really answer your question.

When the rescue personnel arrive, they would be faced with an emergent situation where every minute counted. Rather than employing complex mathematics to calculate the time left, they would use signs and symptoms to determine how much trouble the victim is in and make a guess as to how fast they must move.

What we are talking about here is called "hypoxia" (low oxygen content in the blood). The symptoms and signs of hypoxia are similar to those of alcohol intoxication. The symptoms might include fatigue, lethargy, giddiness, headache, drowsiness, blurred vision, delusions, hallucinations, sleep, coma, and death. The signs would be loss of attentiveness, poor coordination, slowed reaction times, poor balance, rapid breathing, weakness, and finally collapse. These can occur in any combination and progress as your amateur magician consumes more and more oxygen and his hypoxia worsens. These should give you plenty to work with in constructing your scene.

Your firefighters would assess the person to determine how far along in the process he is. If he is giddy and confused, they would have more time than if he is in a coma and barely breathing. The first thing they would do is try to break open the chamber, but I assume that in your scene this isn't going to be accomplished easily. Short of that, they would attempt to bore a hole through which they can pump oxygen and buy some time.

The addition of diabetes to the situation would greatly complicate things, but only if the person is an insulin-dependent diabetic. Diabetics who are insulin dependent manufacture little insulin themselves and must depend on the injection of insulin for survival. Missing a dose can result in a rapidly rising blood sugar level, the onset of diabetic ketoacidosis (DKA), coma, and death.

The symptoms of rising blood sugar and impending DKA are fatigue, shortness of breath, nausea, lethargy, somnolence, confusion, and finally coma and death. The person may become irrational, delusional, maybe combative and angry, and even have hallucinations. As you can see, the symptoms of diabetic ketoacidosis and hypoxia are very similar. Diabetics have been arrested for DUI because they were driving erratically and failed a field sobriety test, only to be found later to have diabetes.

The combination of low oxygen and rising blood sugar is additive so that the symptoms and the danger level progress much faster. This is more pressure for your firefighters and a true ticking time bomb. They now have to get oxygen and insulin to him and have less time to do so.

Perhaps they could open a hole and supply oxygen, but by then he could be too far gone from his diabetes to follow instructions or give himself insulin. The opening would be too small for anyone to get through to help him, and something might prevent them from making the hole bigger. A gas line? Electrical conduit? Steel beam? Wall cave-in?

Cool stuff. Just when it seems to be over, it isn't.

Can Paramedics Determine If an Accident Victim Is Alive by Measuring Liver Temperature?

Q: I read somewhere that paramedics can use some type of apparatus to do a liver test and determine if an accident victim is alive or not. What is this test?

A: Paramedics use vital signs (blood pressure, pulse, breathing, consciousness) to determine if someone is alive, dead, or in transition. If these signs are absent, they begin cardiopulmonary resuscitation (CPR) and ask questions later.

The liver test you refer to is done by the coroner or the criminalists under his direction to aid in the determination of time of death. The apparatus is a thermometer, and it is inserted into the liver to determine the core body temperature, which helps in the timing of physiologic death. It serves no other purpose as far as I know. It definitely has no place or value in the treatment or evaluation of an injured individual.

I can't imagine any situation in which a paramedic would do this—that is, unless he wanted the victim's family to file assault charges against him. Until the victim is pronounced dead by an M.D., he is still alive, and therefore this would be an assault. If the victim lived, it would definitely be an assault.

The duties of paramedics are to support, stabilize, and transport the ill and injured under the direction of the nurse at the base station with whom they have radio contact. The nurse, in turn, works under the direction of the M.D. in the ER where the base station is located. This M.D. would *never* allow anything like this to occur since it has no place in patient care but is, rather, a "coroner's tool."

What Is the Difference Between a Psychologist and a Psychiatrist?

Q: What are the differences, if any, between the training and abilities of psychiatrists and psychologists? Can they both do psychotherapy and prescribe drugs?

A: Clinical psychologists may have a master's degree and a Ph.D. They do not possess M.D. degrees. They can advise, counsel, and provide various types of psychotherapy. They cannot prescribe drugs or oversee medical therapies.

Psychiatrists are medical doctors. They attend medical school and then complete a residency and maybe a fellowship program in psychiatry. In addition to the services provided by clinical psychologists, psychiatrists can prescribe medications, admit and attend patients in the hospital, and perform all the medical interventions of their specialty.

Both can be effective in helping patients with psychologic problems since this depends more often on compassion, understanding, and common sense than on level of training.

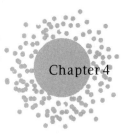

Chapter 4

MEDICATIONS AND DRUGS

What Are the Effects of the So-Called Date Rape Drugs?

Q: What are the major effects of the date rape drugs?

Do they need to be drunk as soon as they are placed in a drink to be effective? For instance, could my villain place one of them in a bottle of water and then appear to freshly open it for someone to drink at a later time?

How aware is the victim after being drugged? I know that there is amnesia afterward, but when you are under the influence, do you know what is happening?

How much should be given to immobilize someone?

Could my villain perform surgery on the victim in this state?

A: The major date rape drugs are Rohypnol (flunitrazepam), Ecstasy (3,4-methylenedioxymethamphetamine), GHB (gamma-hydroxybutyrate), and Ketamine (ketamine hydrochloride).

Ecstasy, GHB, and Ketamine are commonly found at raves—all-night dance parties that attract huge crowds of teens and young adults. The rave culture has its own music, dress, and drug use patterns. Some ravers claim these drugs seem to enhance the rave experience, especially if taken with alcohol.

Rohypnol, GHB, and Ketamine are commonly used in "date" or

"acquaintance" rapes. They are powerful and cause sedation, a degree of compliance, poor judgment, and amnesia for events that occur while under their influence. It is this that makes them effective in date rape situations. A small amount of GHB or Rohypnol can be slipped into the victim's drink in a bar or at a party. She may appear to be no different, but she may leave with her assailant because judgment is impaired and euphoria is enhanced. Only later will she realize that something happened, but her memory of events may be spotty or absent.

With any of these drugs, users may act, talk, and appear normal to those around them. Or they might seem happy, excited, pleasantly sedated, or intoxicated. Or the victim may become "drunk" quickly, develop slurred speech, and, of course, must be put to bed. Or driven home. Or robbed. Or murdered. In any event, she doesn't put up much of a fight. The reaction varies from person to person.

Let's look closer at these drugs:

Rohypnol (street names are Roofies, Roaches, Rope, and Mexican Valium) is a benzodiazepine sedative in the same family as Valium, and it was developed to treat insomnia. Currently, the drug is neither manufactured nor approved for use in the United States, but it is available in Mexico and many other countries. It is manufactured as white 1- and 2-milligram tablets that can be crushed and dissolved in any liquid. The going rate on the street is about $5 a tablet. It takes effect twenty to thirty minutes after ingestion and peaks in about two hours; its effects may persist for eight to twelve hours.

Roofies typically cause sedation, confusion, euphoria, loss of identity, dizziness, blurred vision, slowed psychomotor performance, and amnesia. The victim has poor judgment, a feeling of sedated euphoria, and poor, if any, memory of events. Victims may suddenly wake up or reenter reality hours later with spotty or no memory of what has happened. Rarely, Rohypnol can cause anger and aggressive behavior.

Ecstasy (street names are E, X, XTC, MDMA, Love, and Adam) was originally patented in 1914 as an appetite suppressant, but it was never marketed. It is made in underground labs and distributed in pill or capsule form. It has amphetamine (speed-like) as well as hallucinogenic effects. The user has enhanced sensations and feelings of empathy, a mood lift, increased energy, and occasionally profound spiritual experiences or an equally profound and irrational fear reaction. It may cause increased blood pressure, teeth grinding (bruxia), sweating, nausea, anxiety, or panic attacks. Rare cases of death have been reported from malignant hyperthermia (sudden and marked elevation of body temperature to 106, 108, or above, which basically "fries" the brain).

Now the confusing part. Both MDMA and GHB are sometimes referred to by the slang term Ecstasy, though they are actually very different compounds. The street purchaser doesn't always know which one he is getting.

GHB (street names are G, XTC, E, Liquid Ecstasy, Liquid E, Easy Lay, Goop, Scoop, and Georgia Homeboy) was developed over thirty years ago and was sold as a natural food supplement and muscle builder. It comes as a white powder that dissolves easily in water, alcohol, and other liquids. Currently, it is often found as Liquid E, a colorless, odorless liquid that is sold in small vials and bottles for $5 to $10.

The effects of GHB appear quickly, five to twenty minutes after ingestion, and typically last for two to three hours. It causes loss of inhibitions, euphoria, drowsiness, and, when combined with alcohol, marijuana, cocaine, and many other drugs, increases the effects of these drugs. Many kids use it to enhance the effect of alcohol for a "cheap drunk." Users report that GHB makes them feel happy, sensual, and talkative. They may experience giddiness, drowsiness, amnesia, an increased sense of well-being, enhanced sensuality, and sometimes hallucinations.

Ketamine (street names are K, Special K, Kit-Kat, Purple, and Bump) is a rapid-acting intravenous or intramuscular—and therefore injectable—anesthetic agent that causes sedation and amnesia. It was a common surgical anesthetic agent in the 1970s but fell from favor partly because of its unpredictable hallucinogenic and psychiatric side effects. It is still occasionally used medically and is popular in veterinary medicine as an animal sedative. In fact, the Ketamine that appears on the street is often stolen from animal hospitals and clinics.

A newcomer on the drug scene, it is also available as a white powder or in pill form. It is rapidly absorbed after ingestion or if snorted, which is the most common method of usage. Special K goes for $10 to $20 a dose. When snorted, it takes effect almost immediately and is fairly short in its duration of action—an hour or two.

Many of its effects are similar to Ecstasy, but it also possesses dissociative effects, which means the person separates from reality in some fashion. Often the user experiences hallucinations, loss of time sense, and loss of self-identity. One common form is a "depersonalization syndrome" where the person is part of the activities while at the same time is off to the side or hovering overhead watching the activity, including his or her own actions. This reaction is common with PCP (Phencyclidine, Angel Dust), which was very popular in the 1970s and 80s.

Users call these effects "going into a K hole." I would suspect a K hole is similar to Alice's rabbit hole, where time, space, and perceptions become distorted.

And don't forget the original Mickey Finn or Mickey, a staple in 1940s and 50s detective novels and movies. It was made by combining alcohol with chloral hydrate syrup.

Easy to come by, chloral hydrate is sold as a children's sedative under the name Noctec. A teaspoon assures a good night's sleep—for the child and the parents. However, when mixed with alcohol, it is a powerful sedative. It originally came as a liquid that was added to a mixed drink; now it comes as a soft gelatin capsule as well. Its smell and taste, which is minimal, is easily covered by the alcohol and the mixer of the cocktail.

Since the introduction of barbiturates, chloral hydrate's use as an adult sedative has waned. "Barbies" are more effective and possess fewer side effects. Of course, barbiturates can be mixed with alcohol and lead to the same result. This combination is a common method of suicide.

Now, let's get to your questions.

These compounds are stable and could be added to water, juice, or alcohol hours or days ahead of time. They dissolve easily, and the victim usually has no indication that her drink has been altered.

Even as the drug begins to take effect, the victim is not likely to know she has been drugged, but, rather, feels as if she has had one too many. She is probably happy and euphoric. She may laugh and giggle and be open to persuasion, or she may become very sleepy and lethargic.

Dosing is a problem with GHB and Ecstasy since they are cooked up in garages and basements, but Rohypnol and Ketamine are pharmaceutically manufactured. A triple or quadruple dose of either would likely put the victim out. But a single or double dose might make her compliant, and she would willingly go wherever her assailant suggested. In the scenario you outlined, the victim might willingly participate in sex or other activities, but the pain of surgery would definitely awaken the victim. She may not be able to put up much of a fight or make a great deal of noise, but she wouldn't be very cooperative, either.

Only Ketamine would be strong enough to serve as a surgical anesthetic, and even that would probably require the injectable variety. None of the others are likely to induce coma or complete sedation unless a large dose that could be fatal were administered.

A more realistic scenario might be for the victim to be given a drink spiked with Rohypnol or GHB, enticed to a remote area, and subdued. Then injectable Ketamine could be used as an anesthetic for the surgery.

How Do Drugs Alter the Size of the User's Pupils?

Q: I've read that different drugs affect the size of the pupils in different ways. What are the effects of marijuana, speed, heroin, and some other common drugs on the pupils?

A: The pupils are highly reactive (Figure 7). They rapidly respond to various external and internal stimuli. Enter a dark room, and they dilate (enlarge) to gather more light. Step into the sunlight, and they immediately constrict (narrow) to protect the delicate retina from light damage. Sometimes this reaction can be tricked. We've all heard the warnings regarding direct viewing of a solar eclipse. In this situation the blocking of the sun by the moon tricks the eye into thinking it is darker than it actually is. Light rays from the corona and from the edges of the sun just before and after the total eclipse are stronger than they appear. Staring at the eclipsed sun directly can result in retinal damage.

In addition, through neurological and chemical connections, the pupils are intimately tied to the autonomic nervous system (ANS). The ANS is divided into two subsystems: the sympathetic (flight or fight) and the parasympathetic (feed or sleep). These two subsystems perform a constant balancing act. In an exciting or life-threatening situation the sympathetic side takes control. The heart rate and blood pressure rise, breathing increases, body temperature shoots up, and the pupils dilate. This is the result of a massive outpouring of adrenaline from the adrenal glands. The body is now prepared to fight or run. In a feeding or resting circumstance, the exact opposite occurs. Adrenaline levels are low, as are the heart rate, blood pressure, and body temperature, and the pupils tend to constrict.

Certain chemicals may artificially produce similar reactions.

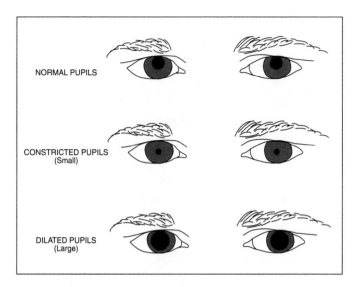

FIGURE 7. PUPILLARY REACTIONS TO DRUGS
Normal pupillary reactions (A) occur to light and stimuli by way of autonomic nervous system. Various drugs also affect their size. "Downers" such as heroin tend to constrict the pupils (B), while "uppers" such as amphetamines tend to dilate them (C).

"Downers" such as narcotics tend to relax and stupefy (no pun intended) and thus constrict the pupils. These include drugs such as heroin, morphine, and barbiturates. "Uppers," or speedlike compounds, are classified as sympathomimetic drugs since they mimic the effect of the sympathetic portion of the ANS. They tend to dilate the pupils. Cocaine, amphetamines, crystal methamphetamine, Ecstasy, and many diet pills do this. Marijuana also tends to enlarge the pupils.

How Safe Is It to Handle Cyanide?

Q: What would happen if a person handling cyanide didn't wear gloves but had limited contact with it?

A: Obviously, what happens is dependent on what exposure occurred, the concentration of the cyanide handled, and the point of exposure. But cyanide is a toxic and very dangerous substance.

Cyanide can absorb directly through the skin and kill you. Gloves would prevent that. If the powder is shaken into the air and inhaled, it will enter the bloodstream rapidly via the lungs and kill you. If it is dissolved in a liquid and the liquid is spilled on the skin or splashed in the eyes, it will kill you.

It takes only a small amount, and even if a doctor was standing right next to you, you would still die.

Bad stuff. Unless you want your character to kill someone, then it's great. But there is no such thing as too much caution when handling it.

Will Food Intake Prevent Alcohol Intoxication?

Q: My character is in a situation where she must drink considerably while minimizing the effects of intoxication. Is there a substance that one can inject or ingest to combat alcohol intoxication (prior to consuming the alcohol)? What about the old adage that a significant quantity of bread will "absorb" the alcohol?

A: Ingested alcohol is absorbed into the bloodstream very rapidly, and as soon as the blood passes through the liver, the liver begins to extract it from the blood and break it down. The level of alcohol in the blood at any given time is a dynamic balance between the rate of absorption from the gastrointestinal (GI) tract and the rate of destruction and elimination by the liver.

Bread does not absorb or soak up alcohol. But any food in the stomach, including bread, will slow the passage of alcohol into the bloodstream and thus lower the blood alcohol level. Alcohol is absorbed at all levels of the GI tract but enters the bloodstream faster from the small intestine, particularly the duodenum (the first part of the small intestine), than from the stomach. Fatty foods and milk tend to slow stomach emptying and thus would hold the alcohol in the stomach longer. The net effect is a slowing of alcohol absorption, so a cheeseburger and a milk shake might be a better pre-binge meal. Of course, drinking less and drinking slower makes the most sense for your character.

How Dangerous Is It to Transport Heroin in a Swallowed Condom?

Q: If you have a "mule" who has swallowed a condom full of heroin, how long before he passes it? How likely is the condom to succumb to digestive fluids and leak?

A: Normal gastrointestinal (GI) transit time (the time required to go from one end to the other—you get the idea) is twenty-four to seventy-two hours, a broad range. The actual transit time varies greatly from one person to another and from day to day in a given individual. In addition to this personal variability, it changes with age, the type of foods eaten recently, any GI diseases that might be present, any medications taken, the level of hydration, and a ton of other factors. Transit time is hard to predict.

That said, the mule would probably pass it in one to three days. Of course, the condoms are visible on an abdominal X ray, so if the customs officer or DEA agent suspects someone, he can easily find the contraband. He then gives laxatives to speed up the transit time and soon has the evidence in hand, so to speak.

The carriers use condoms or other latex, rubberlike containers because the body can't digest them easily, if at all. However, the acids and digestive enzymes found in the GI tract, coupled with the peristaltic motions of the intestines, can weaken a condom and cause it to leak or break. In this circumstance death from absorption of the huge dose of cocaine, heroin, or other drug is typically quick and dramatic. Cocaine and methamphetamine cause seizures, cardiac arrhythmias, heart attacks, and death. Heroin causes a dramatic drop in blood pressure, suppression of respiration to the point of apnea (no breathing), and death.

Can Opium Addiction Make Someone Violent?

Q: I need help. One of my characters has found a hundred-year-old suicide letter. The writer says he has become addicted to opium, his personality has changed, he's become violent and nasty, and he intends to kill himself to keep from burdening his family. My writers' group questioned whether opium would make someone violent. If someone did become addicted to a substance in the late 1800s and had a personality change for the worse, what drug would it have been if not opium?

A: Opium, which is a gummy substance obtained from the opium poppy (*Papaver somniferium*), is a central nervous system depressant. It's the basis for morphine and heroin, and is a "downer." It causes lethargy and sleepiness, slow movements, depression, and in larger doses, coma and death. It is unlikely to stimulate violent or nasty behavior. That said, an opium addict who is undergoing withdrawal, either voluntary or forced, either jailed or unable to resupply himself, can become angry, aggressive, and even homicidal. So, yes, opium can indirectly cause the effects you want.

One other thought: In your scenario it is the letter writer who states that his own behavior has changed. Is that real or imagined? Is there corroboration of this statement from a more reliable source? He's an addict, so his assessment may not be accurate. Maybe he is having violent dreams or hallucinations that he believes are true when in fact he is as gentle as a lamb—and depressed and suicidal. Opium can easily cause these types of delusions.

Another drug choice might be cocaine, which was available during the nineteenth century. Users often become aggressive, short-tempered, and violent. Chronic use can cause paranoia, which can feed the underlying aggressive behavior. This is probably a better choice if it fits your story.

Of course, he could have been addicted to both drugs. For a brief period of time during the nineteenth century, Sigmund Freud and others advocated cocaine as a treatment for opium addiction. Its stimulatory effects were seen as beneficial. After it became apparent that those treated in this manner became addicted to the cocaine, this treatment modality fell from favor. Perhaps the suicide letter or others found with it could mention that he had sought treatment for his addiction but was now despondent that the cure became its own curse.

Another possibility is alcohol, which is common and easily available. Alcoholics often become aggressive, nasty, and even homicidal. And suicidal.

Suicide is common among opium, cocaine, and alcohol abusers, as are accidental deaths from taking too much or combining drugs such as an opiate and alcohol. An interesting twist might be that the letter finder later acquires other evidence that indicate the suicide was perhaps not a serious attempt by the writer to take his own life but rather a gesture or cry for help that went too far. All too often addicts don't know how to ask for help, especially a hundred years ago, and believe that a suicide attempt will get them the attention they need.

Is Ritalin Useful in the Treatment of Attention Deficit Disorder, and How Can It Be Abused?

Q: My character's twelve-year-old son is put on Ritalin for attention deficit disorder. What would be the usual dose? How effective is it likely to be, and are there any side effects? Also, I read that this drug is commonly abused. How? By whom?

A: Attention deficit disorder (ADD) is not uncommon. It goes by several other names, such as hyperactive or hyperkinetic child syndrome and minimal brain dysfunction syndrome. The characteristic symptoms of this disorder are short attention span, distractibility, emotional lability, impulsive actions, and hyperactivity. Learning may or may not be impaired. The diagnosis of ADD is not straightforward and depends more on the presence of several of these symptoms rather than the results of any specific test. Neurologic exams, such as electroencephalograms (EEGs), MRIs, and CT brain scans, are most often normal.

Ritalin (methylphenidate hydrochloride) is effective for many sufferers of ADD. It is given orally twice per day, typically before breakfast and lunch. The typically recommended starting dose is 5 milligrams (mg) twice a day, which is increased by 5 to 10 mg every week until the desired effect is attained. The maximum dose should not exceed 60 mg per day. Ritalin comes in small round tablets of 5 mg (yellow), 10 mg (pale green), and 20 mg (pale yellow). There is also Ritalin SR (white), a 20-milligram sustained release tablet that is taken only once a day in the morning.

Ritalin may lessen or eliminate the symptoms of ADD. Alternatively, one of its many side effects may occur; these include rashes, loss of appetite, nausea, headache, drowsiness, an increase or decrease in blood pressure and pulse rate, palpitations, and even a toxic psychosis, in which delusions and hallucinations may occur.

Yes, Ritalin is a newcomer to the drug abuse crowd. It is ground and snorted and tends to give a rush similar to cocaine or methamphetamine. Many primary schools have policies, stating that any medications taken by students during school hours must be given by the school nurse. The school bullies know this and watch to see which kids visit the nurse each morning to get their daily medications. Then they force the kids to hand them over and use the pills themselves or sell them to someone—kind of like a primary school Mafia.

It is also found in high schools and on college campuses. An unscrupulous doctor or pharmacist can often be found who will prescribe or dispense the drug. In addition, Ritalin is an overprescribed medication (meaning it is given to patients who don't really need it, much as Valium was in the past), and thus there is a lot of it out there on the streets. A ready supply and a growing demand means escalating abuse.

What Is Seasickness?

Q: My novel is set in Victorian Boston. One of my characters, a middle-aged woman, must sail to England. She has severe seasickness every time she gets on a boat. What treatment might her physician suggest to get her through the trip?

A: There were many treatments for seasickness at that time, but none of them worked very well. One reason was that little was known of the physiology of this disorder. One popular theory postulated that it was caused by disturbances in the circulation of blood to the brain, which caused it to become anemic and thus produced nausea, vomiting, and dizziness, the major symptoms of motion sickness.

We now know that seasickness, motion sickness, and space sickness (due to weightlessness) are caused by scrambled signals received by the vestibular system (balance center) of the inner ear. As part of this elaborate system, the semicircular canals are the primary sensors of position and motion. They consist of three canals, each in a 90-degree plane to the other two, similar to the XYZ planes of solid geometry. One loops front and back, one right and left, and the last up and down. The canals are filled with fluid, and the action of gravity on this fluid lets the brain know if it is right side up, upside down, moving in a circle, and so forth.

In a weightless environment these signals are lost because there is no gravity and therefore the fluid is weightless, and no signals are sent. Yet the brain needs these signals for orientation. Without them, vertigo and the other symptoms of motion sickness occur. In moving cars and ships, the fluids slosh around so that the brain receives chaotic and confusing signals, resulting in the same symptoms.

In a report in the March 16, 1901, issue of the *Journal of the American Medical Association,* Dr. Daniel R. Brower offered the following treatment plan: Before the trip one should "avoid excessive fatigue and mental worry," eat lightly, and produce a "free catharsis by means of a full dose of massa hydrargyri, followed at the proper time by a saline purgative." (What he meant by "full dose" and "proper time" was not explained.)

Once this cleansing of the bowels had been accomplished, he suggested adding one teaspoon each of "Potassii Bromidi" (potassium bromide) and "Aq. Menthae Piperitae" (mint or peppermint oil) to water and drinking it three times a day until boarding the ship. Once on board, one should then take 10 to 15 grains (1 grain equals approximately 65 milligrams) of "Chloralamid," lie down, and remain horizontal until the ship was at sea and the effects of the medication had worn off. (He did not comment on what these effects might be.) Then one should "move around on deck to ascertain whether he has obtained his 'sea legs.' " If the seasickness returns, the Chloralamid should be repeated. His last and probably best advice was to "remain on deck as much as possible."

This may be a case of the cure being worse than the disease.

Fortunately for your lady, seasickness tends to resolve over a few days. Of course, "land sickness" can occur with the cessation of the sloshing of the fluids in the canals when the victim steps onto shore. Just when the canals become accustomed to the erratic signals, things return to normal, and once again the system is thrown off. Go figure.

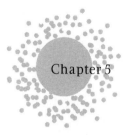

Chapter 5

DISEASES AND THEIR TREATMENT

How Do Heart Disease and Angina Limit My Hero's Activities?

Q: My protagonist is a sixty-seven-year-old man who has heart disease. He has frequent minor heart attacks for which he uses nitroglycerin. He suffers one of his attacks when another man dies at his dinner party. He takes a pill and goes to bed. In the morning I have him resuming his regular activities. Is that feasible?

A: The mistake you're making in terminology is extremely common. Don't feel bad: I see it all the time. Books, newspapers, patients, and TV reporters make the same mistake.

The coronary arteries course over the surface of the heart and supply blood to the heart muscle. A heart attack (myocardial infarction, or MI) occurs when a portion of the heart muscle dies due to complete blockage of one of these arteries (Figure 8). This is a potentially lethal and emergent situation, and requires immediate hospitalization and treatment. Some MIs are silent, meaning there is no pain, while others are associated with mild and brief pain as you describe. However, most often the pain is severe and lasts for hours unless treatment is given. Yes, some people have heart attacks and go on about their business, but this is not the norm.

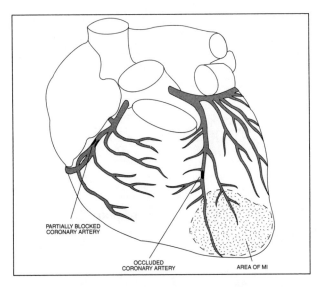

PARTIALLY BLOCKED
CORONARY ARTERY

OCCLUDED
CORONARY ARTERY

AREA OF MI

FIGURE 8. CORONARY ARTERY DISEASE AND ITS COMPLICATIONS
Disease of the coronary arteries can lead to severe illness and death.
A partially occluded coronary artery can lead to angina, a severe and
distressing chest pain. Total occlusion can result in myocardial
infarction (MI), the death of heart tissue.

What you are describing is angina pectoris, "angina" for short.
This is pain coming from the heart muscle due to poor blood sup-
ply because of a partially blocked coronary artery (Figure 8).
Angina does not lead to damage or death of the heart muscle itself.

As you noted, the pill taken for this is nitroglycerin (nitro for
short). It is placed under the tongue (not swallowed), dissolves
quickly, and is absorbed directly into the bloodstream through the
lining of the mouth. Nitro dilates (opens up) the coronary arteries,
which increases the supply of blood and oxygen to the heart muscle and lowers the blood pressure (BP). This, in turn, lessens the
work that the heart must do to move the blood around the body.
The workload that the heart must carry is directly related to the
blood pressure. The higher the BP, the more work—like weight
lifting. Nitro increases supply and lessens demand, thus relieving
the angina pain.

Angina pain is typically a pressure-like heaviness in the middle of the chest, possibly with the spread of the discomfort into the left arm or jaw. Other associated symptoms might include shortness of breath, sweatiness, a cold and clammy feeling, nausea, weakness, and mild dizziness. Anyone who sees your protagonist would know something is wrong. He would likely appear scared, sweaty, and perhaps pale.

An episode of angina typically lasts one to five minutes if untreated. Nitro will resolve it in one or two minutes. After a bout of angina the person may feel tired or fatigued, but in a matter of five to ten minutes he would likely feel okay and be able to go ahead with normal activities.

Obviously, people with angina are at risk for a true MI since any one of the pain episodes can evolve into a full-blown MI. The nitroglycerin would lessen this probability if taken immediately. That is why we tell patients with angina to keep their nitro with them at all times—not in the glove box or a desk drawer or the medicine cabinet but in their pocket or purse so that it is available at a moment's notice.

A diagnosis of coronary artery disease with angina would fit your character's situation well. Throughout your story you could add a note of menace by having him suffer angina attacks whenever he is in a physically or emotionally stressful situation. An uphill walk, an argument, a fight, an emotional reunion or separation, or, as you suggested, the death of a friend or loved one could trigger an attack. Maybe he could have an angina episode and not have his nitroglycerin in his pocket and have to ride it out. This is a situation that would produce great fear. He might later feel foolish for not having his medication with him.

How Would an Allergy to Bee Stings Affect
My Character's Lifestyle?

Q: I have a character with a potentially lethal allergy to bees. How would she live her life? Would she have a Medic-Alert bracelet or an antidote in the fridge? Would bees be attracted to her any more than they would be to a non-allergic person? Would she wear an insect repellent?

A: Bee stings can result in several reactions. In a nonallergic person the sting site would burn and swell, but the reaction remains localized and fades in a couple of days. In allergic persons more severe and painful swelling of the area, which could involve the entire leg or arm, is likely to occur. It would swell like a sausage and be fiery red, painful, and itchy. A worse allergic reaction would involve breathing problems that result from spasm (narrowing) of the bronchial tubes—like a severe asthmatic attack. The victim could die from this without prompt treatment. The worst reaction is full-blown anaphylaxis. Here the swelling and bronchospasm are joined by cardiovascular collapse, which means the blood pressure drops into the basement. Shock and death follow quickly.

Bee sting kits are available. These contain a small syringe of injectable epinephrine (adrenaline), which reverses the allergic effects quickly. The person would then go to an ER for more definitive treatment that would include more epinephrine, if needed, along with an antihistamine (such as Benadryl) and steroids.

The kits can be kept in a purse or pocket. When needed, they are needed "right now," so it's best for allergic people to keep a kit with them at all times, just as heart patients should keep nitroglycerin with them at all times.

The person would live a normal life but would be wise to avoid bees. A walk in the park would require extra vigilance but could be done without much danger. Insect repellent would be useful. It is believed that some perfumes, soaps, deodorants, and other good-smelling products may attract bees, but this is controversial.

I know of no evidence that allergic persons are more likely to attract bees. Clothing color seems to be an issue, but it's not straight-forward. Many people believe that bright colors—reds and yellows—might attract bees, but I recently read of one study that showed black and other dark clothing attracted them, too. Go figure.

What Types of Malaria Exist?

Q: My story is set in Louisiana in the late 1800s and the protagonist suffers from malaria. I understand there are different types of malaria and picture my character hav-ing the variety that never completely goes away but causes slow degeneration (anemia? gradual weakening? eventual death?). What type would that be? Also, do the chills always precede the fever? If the protagonist is given watered-down quinine, would the medicine sup-press the symptoms, and would he then have milder chills and fever? I've also heard of a fever remedy called boneset. Would that be effective against malaria?

A: Malaria was and is one of the world's leading killers. Cur-rently, at least 300 million people become infected each year, and as many as three thousand die each day. Though it is now rare in the United States, it was not uncommon in the swampy areas of Louisiana in the nineteenth century.

Malaria is what we call a protozoan disease. Protozoa are tiny single-celled organisms at the very lowest level of the animal kingdom. Protozoa of the Plasmodium family cause malaria. There are four types: *Plasmodium vivax*, or *P. vivax*; *P. falciparum*; *P. malariae*; and *P. ovale*. The most common type in the southeast United States and South America is *P. vivax*. *P. falciparum* is the most deadly and even with treatment has a mortality rate of 20 percent. For your scenario, *P. vivax* is the best choice.

The life cycle and the infection cycle of malaria are very complex and vary from species to species. I'll focus on what happens in the case of *P. vivax* and try to simplify it.

Malaria and many other diseases are transmitted to humans via a "vector," or carrier. In the case of malaria the vector is the anopheles mosquito. The mosquito itself becomes infected when it bites an infected person. The malarial organisms enter the mosquito with the blood it extracts. They then reproduce and concentrate in the mosquito's saliva. When the mosquito bites someone else, the organisms are injected into the person's bloodstream. From here two developmental cycles occur.

The first is the hepatic (liver) cycle, and the second is the erythrocytic (red blood cell, or RBC) cycle. In the hepatic cycle the malarial organisms injected into the bloodstream make their way to the liver and set up housekeeping in the liver cells, where they reproduce. This is the incubation period, and the victim usually has no symptoms. This typically last for about eight days, but the organisms may remain dormant in the liver cells for months or years. Sooner or later they reproduce, rupture the liver cells, and reenter the bloodstream. Symptoms begin at this stage.

The organisms then enter the RBCs and the erythrocytic cycle begins. They reproduce in the red blood cells and eventually rupture them, return to the bloodstream, infect more RBCs, and this cycle continues. In *P. vivax* this erythrocytic cycle occurs every forty-eight hours, although early in the infection this may be erratic. Eventually, they all seem to get on the same schedule.

Interestingly, the presence of sickle-cell anemia tends to protect those individuals from malarial infection. It may be that the parasite can't reproduce properly in sickled cells. Since malaria is common in many areas of Africa, it is possible that people of African extraction, where most sickle-cell anemia is found, developed this mutation as a survival benefit.

The initial symptoms are like a flu: fever, chills, malaise, headache, muscular soreness and stiffness, poor appetite, nausea, and vomiting. Soon the classic cycle of fever, chills, and rigors (uncontrollable shaking) occurs about every forty-eight hours along with the rupturing of the RBCs and the release of large numbers of the organisms into the bloodstream. Obviously, the continued destruction of RBCs in this fashion leads to anemia. The victim may also appear jaundiced (a yellow hue to the skin). Over time, the liver and/or the kidneys can fail, and death may follow.

Quinine comes from the bark of the cinchona tree, originally found in Peru. The bark was ground and used to treat "intermittent fevers" as early as 1712. In 1820 two French chemists, Pierre Pelletier and Joseph Caventou, extracted quinine from the bark and made a powder of sulfate of quinine that proved to be more effective in treating the fevers than the bark itself.

During the nineteenth century, quinine was the major treatment for malaria. Not a pleasant medicine, it tastes bitter and causes nausea, vomiting, diarrhea, skin rashes, ringing in the ears, and even hearing loss for high-pitched frequencies. Used in smaller doses, as you suggested, it would have fewer of these side effects and would only blunt the symptoms of the disease, as you guessed. Without full and aggressive treatment the malaria would never resolve, and the person would be infected for life. Africa and South America have millions of people who live just this way. Many eventually die of the anemia, liver or kidney failure, or another infection such as pneumonia—victims of malaria are more prone to other infections than the norm.

Boneset *(Eupatorium perfoliatum)*, also known as feverwort, agueweed, or sweatplant, is a flowering plant that was dried and used to make a bitter tea. It causes flushing and sweating, and was used to treat fevers and also as a laxative. Several North American Indian tribes found it useful, and it was adopted from them by European settlers. I know of no evidence that it was effective against malaria. Its use as a folk remedy, both then and now, is due to its ability to cause sweating, which was seen as beneficial. It is not.

What Exotic Diseases Are Prevalent in the Caribbean?

Q: My heroine's daughter returns from a trip to the Caribbean very ill, requiring that she be hospitalized. I thought of severe "turista" and hepatitis as possible illnesses but would prefer something a little more exotic. Any thoughts?

A: Schistosomiasis. Exotic enough?

A mouthful for sure, it is pronounced: shish-toe-so-my-a-sis. It is an infection caused by a trematode (a worm in the fluke family) and there are several species worldwide. In the Caribbean the most likely type would be *Schistosoma mansoni (S. mansoni)*. It is endemic to many parts of the Caribbean, and victims contract it if they swim or bathe in water infected with the parasite. Any freshwater pond or stream can contain *S. mansoni*.

The life cycle of this parasite is complex and interesting (Figure 9). It requires the cooperation of two hosts (human and snail) and the metamorphosis of the organism into several distinct forms. The infective form is called a cercaria. It is a microscopic wormlike organism with a forked tail. It enters the body through unbroken skin that comes in contact with infected water. After entry it transforms into a form called a schistomule and migrates via the bloodstream to the lungs and then to the portal vein of the liver, where it matures into an adult schistosome. Males and females then pair up and migrate to the intestinal lining, where they set up housekeeping, mate, and begin to produce eggs. The eggs either remain in the intestinal tissues or are swept back to the liver. Either way,

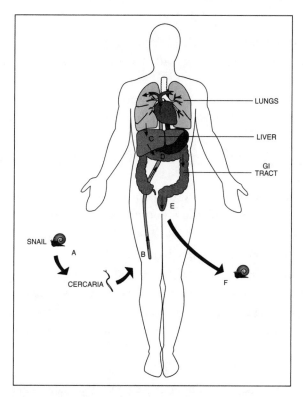

FIGURE 9. THE LIFE CYCLE OF SCHISTOSOMIASIS
Infected snails release cercariae into water (A), and they enter the
human body through unbroken skin (B). The cercariae
transform into schistomules and migrate by way of the
bloodstream to the lungs and on to the liver (C). This form then
matures into schistosomes, which move into the gastrointestinal
tract, mate, and produce eggs (D). The eggs are ultimately
excreted (E). When they once again come in contact with water,
they hatch into their miracidium forms, invade the snail (F), and
transform into cercariae, completing the cycle.

they are ultimately excreted, and when they contact water again,
they hatch into a miracidium, a free-swimming form that moves by
way of cilia (external hairlike structures that function as paddles).
These forms seek out and invade a specific species of snail. Within
the snail they develop into cercariae, and are released into the
water, and the cycle repeats itself.

Within the human body the invasion, migration, and maturation period lasts about four to five weeks. During this time the victim typically has no symptoms, with the possible exception of mild itching for a day or so after initial exposure. Symptoms begin with the egg-laying stage. The most common symptoms are fever, chills, headache, hives or angioedema (puffy swelling of the hands, feet, and face, especially the lips and eyes), cough, weight loss, fatigue, abdominal pain, and diarrhea. Occasionally the diarrhea may be bloody.

Diagnosis is difficult, mostly because schistosomiasis isn't considered. It is often confused with typhoid fever, amoebic dysentery, and other diarrheal or prolonged febrile diseases. Lab tests would show an increase in the white blood cell (WBC) count, particularly an elevation of eosinophils (a type of white blood cell) to greater than 50 percent of all WBCs (a normal level would be 3 to 5 percent). Diagnosis is established by finding the eggs in a stool specimen, from a biopsy of rectal tissues, or by a positive immunofluorescent antibody test.

Once diagnosed, treatment is fairly straightforward: a single dose of Oxamniquine (15 milligrams [mg] per kilogram [kg] of body weight [1 kg equals 2.2 pounds]) and three doses of Praziquantel, (20 mg per kg) given six hours apart. Let's say your character weighs about 120 pounds, or 55 kilograms. She would be given 825 mg of Oxamniquine at one time and three 1200-mg doses of Praziquantel six hours apart.

In your story the young victim could have gone swimming in a pool, perhaps near a romantic waterfall or in a tree-shaded stream. She would return home full of stories and feel completely normal. Six weeks later she could develop the "flu." Fever, chills, cough, and mild diarrhea would suggest such a diagnosis. Her M.D. would treat her with aspirin, fluids, and chicken soup, but she would become worse. More fever and chills, weight loss, and bloody diarrhea could develop. She would be hospitalized and evaluated for hepatitis, amoebic dysentery, and perhaps typhoid. Blood tests, barium enemas, and cultures of her blood would reveal nothing except an elevation of the WBC and eosinophil counts. Liver and kidney studies would be normal. Finally, a stool specimen, sent to the lab to look for amoeba organisms, would show the schistosome eggs, and an immunofluorescent antibody test would be performed on a blood sample. The cute young doctor on whom she has developed a crush would make the diagnosis, treatment would be given, and she would go on with her life, none the worse for wear.

What Are the Symptoms and Signs of Spinal Muscular Atrophy?

Q: I've afflicted a major character in my book with chronic spinal muscular atrophy. The book is set in fifteenth-century Brittany and France. I chose this disease because I wanted one that would waste the character away, not be contagious, and be quite rare, so that no one would know what to do about it.

At the time my heroine meets him, he is in his twenties and his legs have already atrophied. He knows he is going to die as his brother did, but because the progress of the disease has temporarily slowed, he has hope that he has more years to live.

My critique group keeps asking for more symptoms of his suffering, though I do say his strength is going as the wasting and paralysis moves up his body, and he is in pain as it happens.

Does this scenario ring true? What else can you tell me about this rare disease?

A: Yes, your scenario works well, and you have obviously done your research.

Spinal muscular atrophy (SMA) comes in at least three varieties:

1. *SMA I, Infantile SMA or Werdnig-Hoffmann disease*, is apparent at birth and has a rapidly fatal course. The infant has weak, floppy limbs and poor reflexes, and usually dies in the first year. Not suitable for your story.

2. *SMA II, Chronic Childhood SMA*, begins in later childhood and has a slowly progressive course.

3. *SMA III, Juvenile SMA or Wohlfart-Kugelberg-Welander disease*, begins during late childhood and has a slowly progressive course. This is probably best for your scenario.

These are all what we call "lower motor neuron diseases." They affect the neurons (nerve cells) of the lower spinal cord rather than those of the brain. Motor neurons are those involved in movement as opposed to sensation (sensory neurons). Other diseases in this family include amyotrophic lateral sclerosis (ALS, or Lou Gehrig's disease). Stephen Hawking, the brilliant theoretical physicist, is afflicted with ALS.

SMA is an inherited disease, so the fact that your character's brother died from the same disease fits perfectly and adds a note of fear since the character knows what to expect. Of course, in the 1400s absolutely nothing was known about this disease, and it obviously wouldn't have a name. It is very likely that he would be considered a sinner or possessed or otherwise dangerous. At that time religion had a much stronger hold on people's beliefs than did science.

As you noted, the loss of motor nerve stimulation in your character leads to progressive atrophy of the muscles. This is usually more prominent in the larger proximal muscles of the shoulder and hip girdles. The thighs, upper arms, and shoulders become progressively weak and wasted, month by month and year by year.

Pain is not typical with these syndromes since they involve the motor neurons rather than the sensory ones.

The symptoms are simply a progressive loss of strength and

muscle size, beginning in the larger muscles and progressing to the smaller ones. As the weakness advances, loss of coordination and the finer movements of the hands, for example, deteriorate. Hand-writing, drawing, and playing with small objects would suffer. Handling eating utensils or other tools would become awkward and clumsy. Walking would become wider of gait (for better bal-ance) and more shuffling in quality. Trips and falls would be com-mon. The ability to stand, walk, and rise from a chair would become increasingly difficult. Eventually the victim would become chair- or bed-bound and more and more dependent on the help of others for feeding, bathing, dressing, and so forth. Through all this his mind would be completely intact, since this disease does not affect the brain. Of course, depression, sullenness, anger, and thoughts of suicide could appear.

What Type of Bacterial Meningitis Is Most Likely to Infect Adolescents?

Q: I have an unusual question. I am writing a fictional story that is loosely autobiographical. At age twelve, while attending a summer camp, I became very ill, was hospitalized for a couple of weeks, and nearly died. I remember little of the experience but later was told I had had bacterial meningitis and that many of the other kids at camp had the same thing. I want to use this event in my story and would appreciate your thoughts on what this might have been.

A: Meningitis is an inflammation of the meninges, which are the membranes that cover the brain and spinal cord. The most com-mon at age eleven would be viral meningitis (caused by several dif-ferent types of viruses) or bacterial meningitis (caused by either *Haemophilus influenzae* or *Neisseria meningitidis*, both of which are bacteria). The most likely culprit in the scenario you describe would be meningococcal meningitis, which is caused by *N. meningitidis*.

Meningococcal meningitis most commonly occurs in children under three years of age or in adolescents between fourteen and twenty. It can become epidemic in closed communities such as camps, military bases, and schools, particularly where people come from varied parts of the country. Let me explain why this is so.

Many different strains or types of *N. meningitidis* exist. We all carry these and other bacteria in our nasopharynx (nose and throat). We are immune to them, as are most people in our immediate geographic area. After all, we live with them on a daily basis. When we go to another area of the country, we are exposed to people who carry different strains of the same bacteria. We may have no immunity against these strains because we have not been exposed to them on a regular basis and thus have not developed antibodies against them. Alternatively, someone may come into our area from another part of the country and expose us to their particular strain. Either way, we are at risk of developing an infection from this foreign bacterium.

This is particularly true for viruses. How many times have you or someone you know developed a flu or cold after a vacation or trip? When you travel in an airplane and visit other areas of the country or world, you are exposed to viruses that are not part of your normal environment. Since your immunity to these viruses is minimal or absent, you become ill.

N. meningitidis is a common bacterium in our nasopharynx. When people from diverse areas gather, as in a camp or military base, someone may bring in a particularly virulent strain to which many of the group, if not most, do not possess immunity; that is, the carrier is immune, but the other members of the group are not. The bacteria can spread from person to person by direct contact (sharing food or drink or by kissing) or through the air by coughing or sneezing. This sets the stage for those without immunity to develop a throat infection. From the nasopharynx these bacteria can enter the bloodstream, spread to the brain, and become meningitis. As it spreads from person to person, an epidemic of meningococcal meningitis occurs. This is probably what happened to you and your friends.

The incubation period is as short as twenty-four hours, so the epidemic spreads rapidly. By the time the first person becomes ill, many others are already exposed and will themselves become symptomatic in short order.

The major symptoms are fever, chills, sore throat, severe headache, stiff neck, photophobia (irritation of the eyes with exposure to light), generalized aches and pains, and nausea. Since it is an infection of the brain, lethargy, disorientation, confusion, and even coma can occur. This may explain why you remember little of the event.

There are several significant and even lethal complications of this disease. Brain or spinal cord abscesses, pneumonia, meningococcal arthritis, endocarditis (infection of the heart valves), and meningococcemia (a severe infection of the bloodstream that can kill quickly) are not uncommon.

Treatment is with high doses of intravenous penicillin to which the bacterium is very sensitive. Most victims of this illness recover completely with proper treatment.

Is Shock Therapy Effective Treatment for Severe Depression?

Q: I need to know about shock therapy for depression. One of my characters is severely depressed and has tried all the medications. Is shock therapy still done? How is it done? Does it work? What are the complications?

A: Major clinical depression is a common and significant medical problem. It robs the sufferer of all that is good about life. The person is sad and lonely, sees no future, enjoys no one's company, avoids social activities, cries, and often fails to care for himself. In its severest form the person's clothes are dirty: he doesn't bathe and eats poorly, if at all; and his health declines from this personal neglect. The mortality rate in severe depression approaches 15 percent, mostly due to suicide.

Electroconvulsive therapy (ECT) was discovered in the 1930s. Over the years many methods have been used to invoke the convulsions necessary for this type of treatment. Initially, drugs were used and then insulin, which drops the blood sugar to such low levels that a seizure occurs. Finally, electric shock delivered to the brain was employed.

The mechanism of its action and benefit are poorly understood. It seems as though the chaotic electrical activity that rages through the brain during the generalized (grand mal) seizure that the ECT produces somehow alters the mood center of the brain. No one knows for sure, but the results can be dramatic.

In the early years ECT was done without anesthesia so that when the seizures occurred, the recipients would sometimes severely bite their tongues, vomit and aspirate, or even break bones in their extremities from the violent nature of the provoked convulsions.

In 1975 the movie *One Flew over the Cuckoo's Nest* hit the screen and painted a negative picture of ECT. Here it was used as a punitive device, as opposed to a therapeutic endeavor. Currently, it is making a comeback, simply because it works. It is safe and effective as the first line of treatment for severe depression, with response rates of 80 to 90 percent. In people who have failed medical therapy, as in your character, it is effective in 50 to 60 percent of cases. As with any therapy, relapses after ECT may occur.

The procedure is much less barbaric than it once was. The patient is placed on a stretcher, an IV is started, cardiac monitoring electrodes are placed on the chest, and the ECT electrode patches are applied to each side of the head. Either an Ambu bag with face mask is placed over the mouth and nose or an endotracheal tube is introduced into the trachea (windpipe) in order to ventilate the patient during the procedure and until the anesthetic and muscular paralytic agents wear off.

The patient is then given a short-acting general anesthetic and a muscle relaxant, which prevent the outward manifestations of the seizure and thus prevent the tongue biting and bone breaking of the past. Short-acting anesthetic agents used in this circumstance might include 25 to 50 milligrams of Diprivan (propofol) given by IV and repeated as necessary or 2 to 5 milligrams of Versed (midazolam HCL) given by IV and repeated as necessary. Their effects are seen immediately and wear off quickly. Muscle paralytics used might include .10 milligrams per kilogram (1 kilogram equals 2.2 pounds) of Norcuron (vecuronium bromide) given by IV or 1 to 4 miligrams of Pavulon (pancuronium bromide) given by IV. Each of these takes effect immediately. Dosing can be repeated as necessary and wears off over twenty to thirty minutes.

The physician performing the ECT pays close attention to the patient's heart rhythm and airway to prevent complications from aspiration or cardiac arrhythmias. The electrical current is applied to the brain, and the seizure activity is induced. Since the patient is anesthetized and paralyzed, no tonic-clonic jerking, which happens in generalized seizures, occurs.

For severe depression six to twelve treatments are given at the rate of three times a week or longer, until the desired response occurs. Long-term side effects appear to be minimal, if any. In the short term there may be a dulling of cognitive function (thinking and problem solving) for a few days or weeks. There may also be amnesia, which can be retrograde (events that occurred prior to the ECT) or anterograde (events that occur in the period just after the ECT). In either case, these tend to resolve over a few days or weeks.

Besides this treatment being effective, it does not have the long-term problems associated with many of the psychotropic drugs used in the treatment of depression. These medications not only have significant side effects but also may interact with other medications and certain foods.

What Are the Symptoms of a Miscarriage?

Q: I'm working on a scene in the early 1900s with a female character falling ill, probably having a miscarriage. Can you help me get an idea of what a miscarriage would feel like? Severe cramps? Bleeding? Warning signs?

A: A miscarriage occurs when a fetus is no longer viable and the uterus expels it. This may result from many causes. The fetus may be genetically defective so that its full-term survival was impossible from conception; the placenta may be poorly formed or function improperly, resulting in fetal death; the uterus may be scarred from old infections or trauma such as a previous dilatation and curettage (D and C) or abortion and may not be able to support the growing fetus; or a healthy fetus may be injured or killed by trauma or infection. The Hollywood staple is for the woman to fall or be pushed down some stairs or fall from a horse. These and many other types of blunt abdominal trauma may injure or kill the fetus and result in fetal loss.

The symptoms of impending miscarriage include vague or cramping lower abdominal pain, nausea, diaphoresis (sweating), dizziness, and vaginal bleeding. The bleeding may be minimal and spotty, which may occur in pregnancy without impending miscarriage, or it may be brisk and profound. Ultimately, it will become significant and may be associated with "water breaking" if the pregnancy has progressed far enough for a significant amount of amniotic fluid to develop. This would be followed by passage of the fetal and placental tissues. Early on, in a pregnancy that is only a few weeks along, these tissues are amorphous and ragged, looking more like a large clot of blood. After two months or so a formed fetus may be expelled.

A miscarriage may occur fairly suddenly or may stutter along for several weeks, depending on many factors. For example, the woman may experience severe lower abdominal pain, nausea, sweating, weakness, and the passage of blood and tissue over a period of an hour or two. Needless to say, fear and anxiety would accompany this, since this is a painful and potentially lethal event. On the other hand, she might experience several days or weeks of mild cramping and perhaps some spotting. Ultimately, the cramps would become more intense, followed by more significant bleeding and tissue passage.

Afterwards she may bleed a little or a lot, even to the point of exsanguination (bleeding to death). She may develop an intrauterine infection with high fevers and shaking chills, from which she may or may not recover.

One hundred years ago there was little that could be done, and survival depended on how severe the miscarriage was, the degree of blood loss, the occurrence of infections (for which there was no treatment), and luck. She would be put to bed, fed lightly, given warm tea, and sponged with water to relieve any fever. The family would gather, the priest would visit, and the doctor, if there was one, would be summoned, though there would be little he could do.

What Complications of Pregnancy Would Lead to Hospital or Bed Confinement?

Q: I am writing a story that revolves around the pregnancy of an unwed sixteen-year-old. Her pregnancy is difficult in that she experiences nausea, weight loss, and depression. For plot purposes I want her to be confined to bed for the last several weeks of her pregnancy. I

know that several problems can lead to this recommen-
dation by her doctor. What are some of the common
ones I should consider?

A: The four most likely would be premature labor, premature
rupture of the membranes (water breaking), preeclampsia, and
peripartum cardiomyopathy. Let's look at each of these.

Premature labor is when the uterus begins to have contractions
weeks or months before the expected delivery date. If these contractions continue, a premature birth could follow, putting the
child's survival in question. Typically, the contractions begin as
mild and intermittent lower abdominal discomfort, and progress in
frequency and intensity over several days. The expectant mother
may ignore or deny them at first, but if they progress, she will have
to seek medical help. Mild bleeding or spotting may occur.

For premature labor she would be given bed rest, though she
would likely be able to get up for bathroom use, bathing, and eating. The major concern here is that she avoid as much activity as
possible. If the contractions do not subside with these conservative
measures, she would be hospitalized and given intravenous magnesium sulfate (mag sulfate, for short) in an attempt to stop the premature uterine contractions. If this is not successful, delivery,
perhaps via cesarean section (c-section), might be done.

Premature rupture of the membranes is when the water breaks
weeks or months before the expected delivery date. This is more
serious than premature labor. When the membranes break, amniotic fluid is lost, and the "cocoon" within which the fetus lives is
breached. This often triggers full labor, followed by delivery, or
allows a route for infection to enter the uterus. Occasionally, with
proper treatment and good luck, the membranes heal, the amniotic
fluid re-forms, and the pregnancy continues as planned.

For premature rupture of the membranes she would be hospitalized and observed for signs of infection (fever, chills, vaginal discharge) or fetal distress (increase or decrease in the infant's heart

rate or abnormal fetal movements). She would be put at strict bed rest and likely placed on intravenous antibiotics. If she was twenty-eight to thirty-six weeks along, her M.D. would try to buy time with this treatment. If she was thirty-six weeks or more, he might choose to induce labor. Either way, if signs of infection or fetal distress appear, delivery would follow in short order.

Preeclampsia is a common but poorly understood entity. It is estimated that worldwide more than fifty thousand women die from this each year. It is a complex interaction between the mother and the fetus that likely involves the immune system. It is more common with first pregnancies and in women who have diabetes. It is also more common when either the mother or the father was a product of a preeclamptic pregnancy. Curiously, it is less common in women who smoke cigarettes.

Symptoms and signs of preeclampsia include elevated blood pressure; edema (swelling) of the ankles, feet, and hands, and around the eyes; irritability; headache; lethargy; confusion; and protein in the urine. Untreated, it can evolve to eclampsia, which is marked by seizures, coma, severe elevation of blood pressure, and a high mortality rate.

If your young lady developed preeclampsia, she would be hospitalized, put at strict bed rest, given intravenous mag sulfate, and placed on diuretics and other medications to control her blood pressure. Again, this treatment would be continued to buy time until the fetus was beyond thirty-six weeks, and then delivery would be performed.

Another possibility is peripartum cardiomyopathy, a mouthful to say the least. Translation: "Peri" means around. "Partum" means the time of delivery. "Cardio" means heart. "Myo" means muscle. "Pathy" means disease. So peripartum cardiomyopathy means a disease of the heart muscle that occurs around the time of delivery. This is not so difficult after all.

In cardiology there are several different types of cardiomyopathy. Most have in common a weakness of the heart muscle which

leads to the heart's performing poorly as a pump—its main function. The term for this is "heart failure." The weakened heart no
longer pumps the blood through the body as vigorously as it
should, the blood pressure falls to low levels, pressure builds in the
lungs, and the lungs fill with water and become congested—a condition known as "congestive heart failure." Major causes are hypertension (high blood pressure), coronary artery disease with heart attacks,
toxins such as alcohol, and virus infections of the heart muscle.

Peripartum cardiomyopathy is a special form of congestive heart
failure. Its cause is unknown, but it occurs in one of every three
thousand to four thousand pregnancies. For unknown reasons, during the last month of pregnancy and up to five months after delivery,
the mother can develop a weakened heart muscle and slip into heart
failure. The symptoms are shortness of breath, fatigue, and edema of
the legs. The treatment is rest, salt restriction, and diuretics. Sometimes digitalis, which strengthens the heart muscle, is given.

Typically, it begins in the last few weeks of pregnancy and
resolves within a few days after delivery. It worsens with each subsequent pregnancy, and women who suffer this are usually advised
against future pregnancies. There is no known way to either predict or prevent its occurrence.

Over several days to a week your character could gradually
become fatigued, gain several pounds in weight (as the body holds on
to salt in water), become progressively short of breath, develop
swollen ankles, and have to be admitted to the hospital for treatment.

If you want your young lady to be at home, go with premature
labor. If you want her in the hospital, any of these would work.

What Medical Emergency Would Expose a Young Woman's Secret Pregnancy?

Q: In my story a sixteen-year-old girl attempts to hide her
pregnancy from her parents and is successful for several

months. At that time I would like for her secret to be discovered in some way that would be dramatic and threatening to her life. I thought about a miscarriage, but could you suggest any other situations that would put her life in danger? I want her to survive but just be scared.

A: Several situations come to mind.

A miscarriage, as you suggested, would work well. It could occur in a single dramatic event or progress over several days in a stuttering fashion. She could suddenly develop severe lower abdominal cramping pain with bleeding and expulsion of fetal tissues. If she was several months along, a formed fetus would appear. She could collapse and sink into a state of shock, manifested by low blood pressure, a pale appearance with perhaps a bluish tinge to her fingers and toes and around her lips, and a cold, clammy sweat. She would be taken to the hospital emergency room, where IVs would be started and blood and fluids given, and then she would be taken to surgery for an emergency D and C. In this procedure the physician, likely a gynecologist, would remove any retained tissues from the uterus.

Alternatively, she could develop episodic pains, with or without vaginal bleeding or spotting, which would progress until the miscarriage occurred. A visit to the hospital and a D and C would follow. In either circumstance, she would remain in the hospital for a few days but would likely recover completely without any long-term problems—at least, physical problems. Her psychological reactions could be long term and significant.

Another possibility would be an ectopic pregnancy. During fertilization the egg leaves the ovary, finds its way to the mouth of the fallopian tube, and begins to descend toward the uterus. The sperm enter the cervical os (the opening at the end of the cervix) and swim through the cervix and into the uterus. They then migrate up the fallopian tube, where they meet the descending egg. One wins the race, and the actual fertilization takes place within the fallopian tube. The fertilized egg continues downward and into the uterus, where implantation in the endometrium, which lines the uterine wall, occurs and the pregnancy commences.

Sometimes the fertilized egg gets hung up in the fallopian tube (Figure 10). The zygote (the ball of cells that will grow into the fetus) develops normally and continues to enlarge just as it would in the uterus. Early on, the mother's symptoms would be exactly the same as if she had a normal intrauterine (inside the uterus) pregnancy. She may suffer morning nausea, mood swings, breast tenderness, and all the other symptoms of pregnancy. Testing for pregnancy would be positive, and no one would know or suspect that anything was wrong. As the fetus develops and grows, however, the fallopian tube, unlike the uterus, cannot expand to accommodate the enlarging fetus. Ultimately, the fallopian tube ruptures. This may take six to twelve weeks.

The symptoms are similar to a miscarriage except the abdominal pain may be more severe and in the right or left side of the lower abdomen, depending on which tube held the ectopic pregnancy, rather then centralized in the mid portion of the lower abdomen. Vaginal bleeding may be much less dramatic or may not occur at all, since the ruptured fallopian tube would bleed into the abdominal cavity and the uterine os would not likely open to allow passage of blood as it does in a miscarriage.

An ectopic pregnancy typically causes abdominal pain on the right or left side for several days before it ruptures. It is often confused with appendicitis, since the symptoms are similar. A pelvic exam usually reveals a palpable mass in either the right or left lower abdomen in the area of the fallopian tubes and ovaries—an area called the adnexa. If she saw her gynecologist at this stage, he would determine that she had a positive pregnancy test and a tender adnexal mass, and would likely obtain an abdominal ultrasound (a picture of the abdominal contents using sound waves) and make

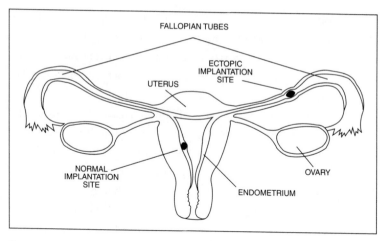

Figure 10. Ectopic Pregnancy
The actual fertilization of the egg by the sperm takes place in the fallopian tube. The resulting zygote migrates to the uterus and implants itself in the endometrial lining of the uterus. Sometimes the zygote does not descend properly but instead hangs up in the fallopian tube, resulting in an ectopic pregnancy. In this circumstance, surgical removal is ultimately required.

the diagnosis of an ectopic pregnancy. Surgery would follow. The affected fallopian tube would be removed. She could still have future pregnancies since the other tube, the ovaries, and the uterus would remain intact.

If she ignored or denied the abdominal pain, it would progressively become more severe and more frequent, but vaginal bleeding or spotting would be unlikely. Eventually, tubular rupture would occur.

Another scenario is that her fear of discovery would lead her into the hands of an unlicensed and unscrupulous clinic where abortions are done, no questions asked—for a hefty fee, of course. Here an unqualified physician or nurse or someone with no medical training at all would perform a makeshift D and C using improper equipment and with poor, if any, sterile technique. The life-threatening complications that might follow are many and severe.

She could continue to bleed from trauma that occurred during the procedure or from retained tissues, if the D and C was incomplete. Pain and bleeding would continue over several days, she would become progressively weaker and more anemic, and her secret would likely be discovered.

She could suffer a perforation of the uterus, a common occurrence in the days of coat hanger abortions. Here, the instrument used to clean out the unwanted pregnancy pushes through the uterine wall and into the abdomen. The uterus is actually perforated quite easily, and physicians performing therapeutic abortions or D and C's are very cognizant of this fact and take great care to avoid this complication. This is a very painful event and leads to severe bleeding and shock. Death is common, since the uterus tends to bleed a great deal when damaged in this manner. Emergency surgery for repair or removal of the uterus would be lifesaving.

She could survive the abortion only to develop an infection several days later. Infections within the uterus are particularly treacherous. The uterus has little capacity to contain infections, and, thus, any bacterial organisms introduced into the uterine cavity by improper sterile technique quickly enter the bloodstream and lead to septicemia (bloodstream infection) and septic shock. Septic shock occurs when the toxins of the bacteria cause severe derangements in the cardiovascular controls of blood pressure and the ability of the body's tissues to use oxygen. The symptoms and signs of septic shock include low blood pressure, high temperatures, shaking chills, confusion, disorientation, and ultimately death. This type of infection has a high mortality rate. Surgical removal of the uterus, high doses of antibiotics, intravenous steroids, and drugs to support the blood pressure are needed if survival is to be realized (dopamine, epinephrine, and Dobutamine are commonly used intravenous agents for this purpose).

What Is the Gulf War Syndrome?

Q: I need some information about the Gulf War Syndrome for a short story I am writing. Everything I've read is confusing, and there seems to be a great debate as to whether it is real or not. Is it? What causes it, and how does it affect the people who have it? Is there any treatment for it?

A: Your confusion is justified. Even the experts argue over whether it is real and, if so, what its causes are. It is a broad and complex subject, and our understanding of the syndrome is in a state of evolution.

The controversy began when many members of our military who returned from the Persian Gulf War began to exhibit unusual symptoms. The most common were fatigue, headaches, memory loss, insomnia, various rashes, swelling and burning of the feet and hands, joint pain and swelling, chronic cough, muscular weakness, loss of coordination, numbness and tingling in their extremities, rectal bleeding, and cardiac arrhythmias with palpitations. This constellation of symptoms became known as the Gulf War Syndrome (GWS).

In medicine the term "syndrome" refers to a group of signs and symptoms that occur together often enough to be recognized as a distinct entity but for which no causal or physiologic relationship has been established. If a man and a woman are walking down the street holding hands, it doesn't mean they are married. In a syndrome the signs and symptoms hold hands, but marriage or any other relationship between them has not been scientifically established. This is the case with GWS.

The cause of GWS is unknown. Some feel it is entirely psychosomatic, while others suggest it is from chemical or biologic weapons used by the Iraqi military or it is the result of our destruction of their chemical weapons bunkers, which released the agents into the air and exposed our troops to the toxic vapors. Still others believe it is related to the vaccines against anthrax and botulinum that our soldiers received or perhaps to the pyridostigmine bromide pills that were given to counteract the effects of many known chemical weapon compounds. The most likely explanation may be a combination of all these. That is, the toxic symptoms may result from a mixture of vaccines and medicines that the soldiers were given and the chemical and/or biologic agents to which they were exposed.

Toxic chemicals that the Iraqi military possessed at that time include sarin, Soman, Tabun, VX, hydrogen cyanide, cyanogen chloride, mustard gas, thiodiglycol (a precursor chemical of mustard gas), and Lewisite. Possible biologic agents include botulinus toxin and anthrax.

Sarin, Soman, Tabun, and VX are powerful neurotoxins that act quickly and damage the neurologic system of those who are exposed. Since many of the symptoms of GWS are neurologic in nature, these chemicals could easily be involved. Mustard gas, thiodiglycol, cyanogen chloride, and Lewisite can damage the skin and lungs. The botulinus toxin and anthrax can cause severe neurologic defects. The vaccines mentioned above as well as pyridostigmine bromide have neurologic side effects.

Unfortunately, a great deal of what is believed, suggested, or speculated to be the cause of GWS has little if any scientific support—not yet, anyway. Research in this area is ongoing. While we await a better understanding of this syndrome, no cure or effective treatment is available.

Part II

Methods of Murder and Mayhem

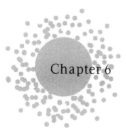

THE EFFECTS OF GUNS, KNIVES, EXPLOSIVES, AND OTHER WEAPONS OF DEATH

Can a Stun Gun Serve as a Murder Weapon?

Q: I'm working on a story that requires one man to kill another while both are in a crowd of people. My thought is that the killer uses a stun gun. While these devices are not supposed to be fatal, is it possible that death could result from the application of a longer-than-usual dose of electricity if the victim has a heart condition or pacemaker?

A: Interesting question.

You are correct in your assumption that stun guns are nonlethal and would result in the death of a normal, healthy adult only in the rarest of cases.

Stun guns and TAZERs deliver a high-voltage, low-amperage shock—usually around 50,000 volts, but some deliver up to 300,000 volts. This causes violent contractions of the muscles and is very painful. Most people collapse to the ground and writhe in pain. Some people are tough and can yank out the TAZER electrodes or knock the handheld stun gun from the attacker's hand. Individuals who are larger, angrier, or on certain drugs such as PCP or methamphetamine would be more likely to overcome the effects of the electric current.

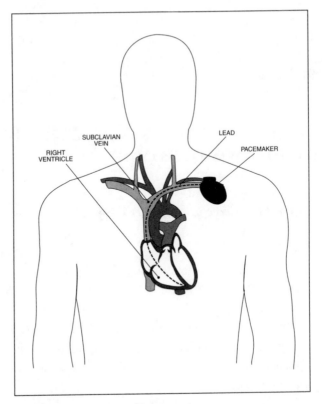

FIGURE 11. CARDIAC PACEMAKER
A permanent cardiac pacemaker, a device to help regulate the heart's rhythm, is placed beneath the skin near the clavicle and is connected to the heart by leads that pass through the veins and into the right ventricle. It serves as a safety net to prevent dangerously slow heart rates.

A pacemaker consists of a pulse generator (the device itself) and leads (wires) that connect the pacer to the heart (Figure 11). Pacers are typically placed just beneath the clavicle (collarbone) and are visible as a watch-dial-sized lump on the chest wall. The pacing leads are passed through the subclavian vein, which lies just beneath the clavicle, and advanced through the superior vena cava into the right side of the heart, where they are wedged into the lower tip of the right ventricle. The leads are then attached to the pulse generator.

The electrical current from a stun device would permanently damage the pacemaker only if it was applied directly over the pulse generator unit itself. This could fry its electronics. A stun gun would have to be held against the chest or the TAZER wires would have to penetrate the skin directly over the pacer for this to occur. If the charge was applied anywhere else on the body, it would be unlikely to harm the pacer itself.

That said, the current could interfere with the sensing function of the pacer in such a way that the pacer would think the heart was beating when it wasn't. A pacer is a demand device, which means it reads the electrical current of the heart and fires only when the heart doesn't. If the heart beats normally, it simply sits and watches. An electrical current could be sensed by the pacer as cardiac activity, and thus the pacer would do nothing.

However, most people with pacers are *not* what we call "pacer dependent." Pacer dependent means that the native heart rhythm is absent or very slow, and without the pacer, the person's heart rate drops to very low levels—thirty beats per minute or less—and death could ensue. Most people have pacers as a safety net for *intermittent* slowing of the heart rate. In this case, interfering with the pacer's sensing function would not be lethal since these patients have a sufficient native rhythm to survive.

A stun device could kill someone with a pacer, but it's unlikely.

As for someone with heart disease, if the person had coronary artery disease or some form of dangerous cardiac rhythm for which he was taking medication, the pain and shock of the attack could precipitate a heart attack or a fatal arrhythmia. Pain, shock, fear, and anger cause the release of adrenaline from the adrenal glands into the bloodstream. This causes an acute increase in heart rate and blood pressure, which could lead to a heart attack or could precipitate fatal changes in heart rhythm.

If your killer knew that your victim had a cardiac history or a "bad heart"—maybe he has daily angina attacks or uses nitroglycerin frequently during physical or emotionally stressful situations—

he could reasonably expect that a TAZER or similar attack might cause the death of the victim. If you set up this background, your method of murder is completely plausible.

What Happens to the Victim of a Stun Gun Attack?

Q: In my current book a character gets hit by a stun gun. What will happen? Will she be unconscious? When will she be able to get up? Will she remember being hurt?

A: Stun guns are handheld contact devices that require the user to place the business end against the attacker's or victim's skin, while TAZERs are handheld projectile devices that fire a pair of darts attached to the hand device by wires. The darts penetrate the skin, even through some clothing. The length of the wire in most commercially available devices is about fifteen feet.

Either will deliver a high-voltage, low-amperage charge that paralyzes the victim by contracting all his muscles. The voltage varies from type to type over the range of 50,000 to 300,000 volts. In some TAZER devices the initial charge will last five to ten seconds and be followed by a series of shorter charges up to about thirty seconds in total duration. This varies by device and manufacturer.

The victim isn't permanently harmed but may require several minutes to recover from the jolt.

The victim will typically drop to the ground, and as the muscles contract, her back will arch and her limbs will convulse as in a seizure. We call these tonic-clonic motions. She may cry out or moan but will not likely be able to make any purposeful movements such as standing, running, or crawling. After several minutes she would be normal once again—perhaps a little more wary but able to perform all physical movements and activities. There should be no residual impairment.

The victim is not unconscious and would probably remember everything, perhaps in great and painful detail.

Will a Stun Gun Shock Others Who Are in Contact with the Victim?

Q: I have a scene where a character who feels no pain is down on the ground being beaten by guards who have nightsticks and stun guns. During the fray one of the guards hits him with his stun gun. If the guard using the stun gun is touching the man, would he be shocked by the electrical charge as well? And would the other guards who are also touching him be shocked, too?

A: The answer is yes to both.

Anyone in contact with the person who is receiving the current will also get the shock. That is why during cardiopulmonary resuscitation (CPR) we yell "clear" before we push the button that releases the current. You have seen this on ER, I'm sure. Otherwise, the person doing the chest compressions, taking a blood pressure, or touching the patient for any reason would also be shocked by the defibrillator current.

Today, many patients have implantable defibrillators (basically a paramedic in a box): this is a device placed beneath the skin of the chest and attached to the heart by electrode wires. These devices monitor the patient's heart rhythm, and when a potentially lethal abnormal rhythm occurs, they deliver a shock to the heart internally, which hopefully restores the rhythm to normal. People touching the patient at the time of discharge will feel a mild shock—nothing harmful or painful but noticeable.

What Would a "Bang Stick" Wound Look Like?

Q: If someone used a "bang stick," like those used against sharks, as a murder weapon, what would the wound look like? Where is the most lethal place to aim it?

A: A bang stick is basically a stick with an explosive charge at its end. The charge is typically a shotgun shell. These devices are used as a defense against sharks and for alligator hunting. The business end is pressed against the target and fired. In some, the shot (lead pellets) are left in the shell so that it acts like a shotgun, while in others the shot is removed and the killing force is the concussive force of the exploding gunpowder.

The wound would be of the contact variety (see the later question, What Does the Wound from a Close-Range Gunshot Look Like? in "The Police and the Crime Scene" section). If the pellets are present, the wound would be as if a shotgun was placed in contact with the skin and fired. The wound would be a combination of the expanding gases, which would rip the skin in a stellate (star-like) pattern, and the shot, which would penetrate into the tissues and cause widespread destruction.

If no pellets are present, the wound would be from the expanding gases alone. The resulting configuration would depend on where the contact was made. If it was over a bone, such as the skull, the explosive gases would expand laterally and rip the tissues into the classic stellate wound. If it was over softer tissues, such as the abdomen, the wound might still appear stellate but would tend to be deeper and less widespread.

The best location to assure the death of the intended victim would likely be against his temple or his neck, where his carotid artery or jugular vein could be injured.

Is a Blow to the Head More Deadly in a Heart Patient?

Q: In my story an elderly man gets hit over the head with a cane. He falls and dies, either from the blow to the head or from his bad heart. Is it feasible that one good blow would kill a man with a bad heart? Would there be a lot of blood around? I'm hoping not, since I would prefer a fairly neat scene.

A: It is indeed possible to die from a single blow to the head with a cane or any other object, especially if the victim is elderly. Older people are especially prone to skull fractures from falls or blows to the head since their bones are more brittle. But even without a fracture, an intracranial bleed (bleeding in or around the brain) can cause death.

Death from an intracranial bleed could occur almost immediately or at a slower rate, depending on the force of the blow, the area of the brain injured, and the swiftness and volume of the bleed. You could almost guarantee death if the victim was not found for several hours and the intracranial bleed was extensive.

An assault of any kind on a person with significant heart disease could precipitate a heart attack or sudden death from a cardiac arrhythmia, which would be caused by the outpouring of adrenaline from the fear and pain that would accompany such an attack. You don't really need that here since the blow alone could do the victim in.

Blows to the head often lacerate (cut or tear) the scalp, which typically bleeds profusely. However, many result in only a bruise or abrasion of the scalp with little if any external bleeding. Either way, an extensive intracranial bleed can occur and lead to death, so it is reasonable for you to have a "fairly neat scene."

Will Ground Glass in Food Kill a Person?

Q: I'm writing a story about an abused wife who decides to kill her husband by feeding him ground glass from a saltshaker. How much would it take to do that? Would it have to go on over time? What would his symptoms be? Would it speed things up if the husband had an ulcer?

A: First the bad news. This is unlikely to work.

The glass would have to be very finely ground, or the victim would notice it as he ate. As we chew, we sense even tiny pieces of gravel, sand, glass, gristle, and so forth. Salt dissolves but glass doesn't, so the food would seem gritty unless the glass was ground into a powder. But very fine glass is unlikely to cause any lethal damage to the GI tract. It would be more of an irritation, with minor bleeding if any at all. If you could get the victim to eat coarser glass, such as crushed instead of ground, the glass shards would damage the stomach and intestine and could cause bleeding.

This works with dogs because they don't really chew their food, and they are accustomed to biting through bones and gristle, and they wouldn't know what the glass was anyway. They simply swallow the larger pieces of glass that do the damage, then go off somewhere and slowly bleed to death. A person would know something was wrong with the food, and if not, he would go to a doctor about the bleeding.

Even with coarser glass, the bleeding would probably not be massive or life-threatening but slow and lead to anemia and fatigue. The stools would become black from the blood, and the victim would see a doctor. Yes, an ulcer would make this worse since he would have two points for potential bleeding, but only the ulcer would have the potential to cause severe life-threatening bleeding. I doubt the ground glass would damage the underlying ulcer enough to cause a severe bleed.

Now, the good news.

If your victim had a serious heart condition such as coronary artery disease (CAD) and had had several heart attacks (myocardial infarctions, or MIs) in the past and now has ongoing angina (chest pain from the heart due to poor blood supply, usually felt as a tightness or squeezing sensation), then the anemia from the slow bleed might lead to a heart attack that could kill him.

In CAD the arteries that supply blood to the heart are narrowed from atherosclerosis. This means that the blood that reaches the heart muscle is reduced by these blockages. Anemia is a condition characterized by reduced red blood cells (RBCs) in the blood. It is the RBCs that carry oxygen, and so in anemia the blood carries less oxygen.

If these two entities occur together, not only does the heart muscle have less blood flowing to it from the obstructed arteries but also the blood it does get has less oxygen—a dangerous combination. We see this a lot. A patient with CAD and mild angina may become very unstable and even suffer a heart attack or die if he develops anemia from a bleeding ulcer or from some other cause.

As the anemia progresses, his angina would get worse, and since he's an abusive jerk, he might not go to his doctor. He would develop progressive and frequent angina attacks, any one of which could blossom into a full MI and kill him.

His M.D. might sign the death certificate since the wife would say her husband had had worsening of his angina, wouldn't go to the doctor, and finally clutched his chest and fell over dead. This way no autopsy would be done, his anemia and his irritated glass-filled GI tract would never be seen by the M.E., and her life would go on.

So the ground glass could work in your story, just not directly.

How Long Does It Take to Smother Someone with a Pillow?

Q: My victim is killed by suffocation—a pillow over the face. How long would this take? She is an elderly woman and not especially strong. She is in a nursing home because of two broken legs suffered in a car accident. I've written this with the assumption that it would be a quick means of killing her. Then I saw somewhere that it can take as long as ten minutes to kill someone this way. So what's the story? Do I have to start over?

A: No, you don't have to start over. An elderly lady would die in two to five minutes and probably toward the lower end of this range. A younger, stronger victim might be able to put up a good fight so that the suffocation would be intermittent; that is, he or she might knock or push the pillow away several times and be able to grab a gulp of air. He would be able to continue this until the oxygen level in his blood dropped sufficiently and he became weak, lost consciousness, and died. Your elderly lady would struggle but probably wouldn't be strong enough to dislodge the pillow, even for a gasp of air. This is particularly true since she has two broken legs and thus would not be able to get much leverage.

Her struggles, as well as the fact that she would be extremely frightened, would lead to rapid consumption of the oxygen in her bloodstream so that death would occur more quickly. Also, an elderly victim such as yours would likely have at least some degree of heart and lung disease, and these would make her tolerance for lack of oxygen even less. Two to three minutes would probably be it.

She would die from cardiopulmonary arrest (the heart stops). If she showed no signs of external injury, her death could be judged to have been natural by her family M.D., since elderly persons frequently die in their sleep—especially in nursing homes after auto accidents. Her private M.D. might assume she had a fatal heart attack or a pulmonary embolism (PE). A PE is a blood clot that travels from the legs or pelvis to the lungs. This is a common cause of death in bedridden patients and in those who have suffered injuries to their lower extremities. Your elderly lady would have both of these risk factors for PE. Her M.D. might sign the death certificate, and that would be the end of it.

But if the M.E. performed an autopsy, he would likely see the characteristic petechial hemorrhages (red dots and small splotches from broken microscopic capillary vessels) in the conjunctivae of the eyes (the pink part). These are found in smotherings and in both manual and ligature strangulations. If he did, a homicide would be suspected.

How Does an Ice Pick to the Back of the Neck Kill?

Q: In my story, a killer shoves an ice pick into the back of a guy's neck, right under the skull, and kills him instantly. Does this work? How?

A: Since life depends on an intact communication between the brain and the body, any injury to the spinal cord in the cervical area is potentially lethal. If an ice pick or knife blade is forced between two of the neck bones (cervical vertebrae) and slices or macerates (chews up) the spinal cord, death is fairly well assured. The cervical portion of the spinal cord is divided into eight levels, which corre- spond to the eight cervical vertebrae. They are designated C1 through C8.

Though damage to any level of the cervical cord could do the trick, the higher the better. Why? The levels between C3 and C5 control respiration, so any injury at or above this level would shut down breathing and lead to death.

Your killer could best accomplish his deed by insinuating his

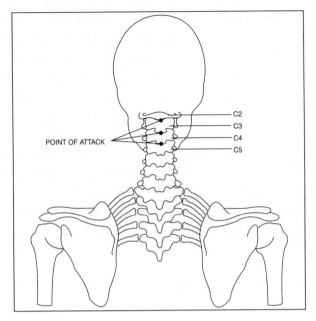

FIGURE 12. THE CERVICAL SPINAL CORD
The brain is connected to the body by way of the spinal cord.
Many vital bodily functions depend on this communication
remaining intact. For any assailant the upper cervical segments
represent the most lethal areas to attack. A sharp instrument thrust
between C2 and C3 would functionally disconnect the brain from
the body and lead to almost instantaneous death.

weapon between the second and third cervical vertebrae (Figure
12). The entry point would correspond with the small hollow
depression in the back of the neck that is just below where the
skull joins the neck. A cut here would anatomically and functionally separate the brain from the spinal cord and, thus, the body.
Think of it as a localized guillotine, a cutting of the spinal cord
without completely removing the head. The effect is the same.

With a transection (cutting) of the spinal cord, all the body's
muscles would immediately become flaccid (limp), and the victim
would drop to the floor. He would be unable to speak or breathe
because the nerves to the diaphragm, which arise from C3 through
C5, would be interrupted. Also, with the loss of enervation to the

body, the blood vessels would rapidly dilate (open up), causing the blood pressure to drop, and shock, unconsciousness, and death would follow.

Would the victim be conscious for a few seconds? Possibly, but he would be as flaccid as a scarecrow, unable to move, speak, breathe, or cry for help. Death would be as immediate as it could be.

What Are the Most Lethal Wounds That Can Be Made with a Knife?

Q: In my story, a right-handed murderer with a very sharp six-inch blade kills a man with one "slice." I know that it's possible for the victim to go into shock and die right away. What I don't know is what the knife has to cut in order to get that result. What would the coroner's report say was the cause of death?

A: I assume from your question that you want the victim to die fairly quickly. There are several possibilities.

A professional assassin can maneuver a blade between the cervical vertebrae (neck bones) and slice the spinal cord in one movement. Usually the attack comes from behind. The assassin slaps a hand over the victim's mouth and thrusts the blade into the back of the neck, slipping it between the bones. The victim goes limp, falls, and dies almost instantly.

From a similar position the killer can draw the blade across the victim's neck, cutting through the carotid arteries and the trachea (Figure 13). Since the carotid arteries supply blood to the brain, the victim dies quickly, and the cutting of the trachea below the vocal cords prevents the victim from crying out. This is what happened to Nicole Brown Simpson.

A thrusting stab wound to the heart is lethal most of the time and fairly quick. The same can be said for the lungs if a major

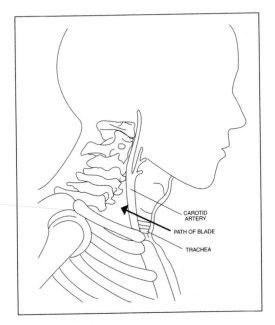

FIGURE 13. THE ANATOMY OF THROAT SLASHING
A knife drawn across the throat can sever the trachea
(windpipe) and the carotid arteries. Death is almost
immediate.

artery is severed. But people often survive stab wounds to the chest
and even the heart, and would, of course, be able to call for help.

A slashing or stabbing wound to the abdomen might work if
the aorta or vena cava was sliced. The problem is that both lie along
the back of the abdomen, and a six-inch blade might not reach them.
It could, though, if the attacker was strong, thrust the knife deeply,
and then made a sweeping motion with the blade. Death would take
several minutes since it would require the victim to bleed to death.

The cervical spinal cord cut, the throat slashing, or the stab to
the heart are the most effective ways and have the highest likelihood of killing the victim.

The coroner or M.E. would be able to determine the cause of

death without difficulty. The cervical cut would be called "transection of the spinal cord at the cervical level." The throat slashing would be termed "transection of the carotid arteries." The stab to the heart would lead to blood filling the pericardium (the sac around the heart), which would compress the heart and interfere with its function. This would be called "death due to pericardial tamponade secondary to a penetrating knife wound." The abdominal stab would result in "death due to exsanguination secondary to a penetrating abdominal knife wound with perforation of the aorta" or vena cava or both.

Gruesome, huh?

What Structures Must Be Injured to Make a Stab Wound to the Back Lethal?

Q: The scenario is for the sleuth to go into the office and find her boss dying with a letter opener lodged in his back.

Is there an artery in or near the lungs? If a victim is stabbed in the back and this artery is hit, would he then literally drown in his own blood? Would the victim be able to speak and give the sleuth the inevitable cryptic clue? If no artery is hit, would the stab wound in one lung be enough to kill him?

A: Let's review a little anatomy and physiology first. Our lungs are designed for gas exchange. This is simply the loading of oxygen into the blood and the removing of carbon dioxide and other toxins from the blood. To do this, the blood and the air must come into close contact with each another. The lungs allow this to happen by having billions of microscopic air sacs and billions of tiny blood vessels that surround these sacs.

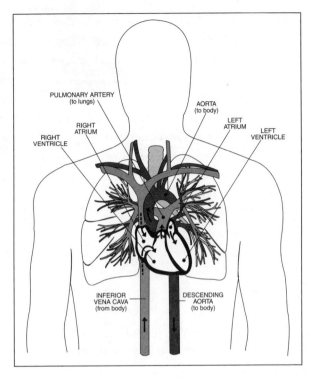

FIGURE 14. THE CIRCULATION OF THE BLOOD
The systemic and pulmonary circuits work as one continuous
circulation system to oxygenate the blood and deliver it to all parts
of the body. Blood from the body flows through the superior vena
cava (upper body) and inferior vena cava (lower body), the right
atrium, the right ventricle, and out the pulmonary artery to the
lungs. After collecting oxygen, it flows through the pulmonary
veins, the left atrium, and the left ventricle, where it is pumped to
the body via the aorta.

The basic circulation system of the body is divided into the systemic and the pulmonary circuits (Figure 14). The systemic circuit
is the left ventricle pumping blood out the aorta and into the various arteries of the body, ultimately reaching every organ and
nook and cranny, and then the blood's return via the veins to the
right side of the heart. The pulmonary circuit is the right ventricle pumping this blood into the pulmonary arteries, which con-
tinually divide into smaller and smaller vessels and spread to all

parts of the lungs like a fan. After the blood collects oxygen, it flows through the pulmonary veins into the left side of the heart and the left ventricle.

This points out two facts important to your question: First, the entire volume of blood in the body flows through the pulmonary circuit continuously. This is necessary since the lungs are the only means available to load vital oxygen into the blood. Second, the lungs, like every other organ in the body, receive a portion of the systemic blood flow. This is the oxygenated arterial blood that keeps the lung tissue itself alive. Thus, the organs known as lungs are extremely vascular (loaded with blood vessels—arteries, veins, and capillaries) and bleed profusely when injured (Figure 15).

Now back to your question. A penetrating wound to the lung as occurs in stabbings and gunshots would result in bleeding into the lung and then out the mouth and nose. The blood coming from these orifices would be bright red and frothy since it is mixed with the air flowing in and out of the lungs as the victim struggles for breath. As the lungs fill with blood, the victim would literally drown in his own blood. The injured lung may or may not collapse, which would only add to the victim's struggle to breathe.

The victim would be able to speak as long as he could move air in and out of his lungs, so he would be able to give the sleuth the telltale clue. If the sleuth was savvy, he might roll the victim onto the side of the injury, using gravity as an ally.

For example, if the victim was stabbed in the left lung and lay on his right side, the blood from the injured left lung would follow the dictates of gravity and flow from the left bronchus (the main airway off the trachea to the left lung) into the right bronchus and then into the right lung. Thus, the "good" lung would fill with blood, and the victim would now have both lungs in trouble and would die more quickly. If your sleuth rolled him onto his left side, gravity would tend to keep the blood in the already injured left lung, and the uninjured right lung would not fill with blood and would continue to function normally. This maneuver might

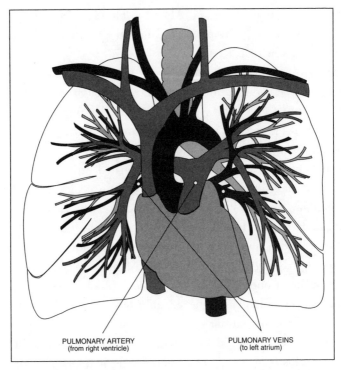

PULMONARY ARTERY
(from right ventricle)

PULMONARY VEINS
(to left atrium)

FIGURE 15. THE BLOOD SUPPLY TO THE LUNGS
The lungs are very vascular, receiving and oxygenating the entire blood
volume by way of the pulmonary circuit. Additionally, they receive a
portion of the oxygenated systemic blood. Any penetrating wound to the
lungs will bleed profusely.

save the victim's life or at least prolong his life so that the needed
clue could be obtained.

What Noises Are Made by Victims of Stabbings or Gunshots to the Neck?

Q: My character needs to walk by a room with an open
door and be drawn in by a hissing or gurgling noise to
find a corpse. Would this type of noise occur if the vic-

tim was shot in the neck? How long might the noises continue after shooting?

A: The short answer is yes.

A gunshot wound (GSW) or any other type of penetrating wound (knife, arrow, ax, machete, and so forth) could produce these sounds if and only if the wound was in the lung itself or one of its airways. The sounds you describe require air moving through a liquid such as blood. Think of a bellows being pumped into a thick liquid, which is exactly what is occurring.

Drowning victims and persons suffering pulmonary edema (literally, lungs filled with water) from heart failure or toxic exposure (such as chlorine or another irritative gas) or certain other processes sound the same way. Again, the sound is that of air bubbling through a liquid regardless of the underlying cause.

A GSW or stab wound to the throat or through the chest into the lung could produce this. Blood would flood the airways (trachea and bronchial tubes), and the movement of air in and out as the victim attempted to breathe would produce a bubbling or gurgling sound. Obviously, these sounds would require that the victim still be alive and trying to breathe when the person walked by the room. He might hear the victim's last breaths and then would find a corpse.

The time lapse from wound to death is extremely variable and depends on the nature, location, and depth of the wound plus the age, fitness, and health of the victim, with the former factors being more important than the latter. This gives you free rein to have the victim die in minutes or hours after the injury.

Can Someone Who Has Been Stabbed in the Neck Speak?

Q: Is it possible for someone shot or stabbed in the neck to utter a few intelligible words before expiring?

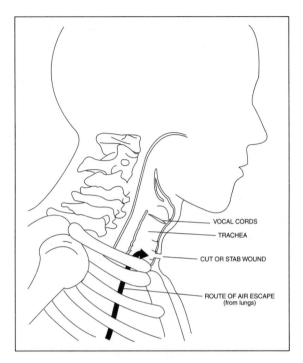

FIGURE 16. ANATOMY OF A SEVERED TRACHEA
Sound requires that air in sufficient volume move across the
vocal cords. A slash wound to the trachea (windpipe) below the
vocal cords allows air to escape before reaching the cords,
rendering speech impossible.

A: Yes, unless the larynx (voice box) or vocal cords are damaged or
the trachea is severed below the larynx or vocal cords. The larynx
is the Adam's apple, and the vocal cords stretch across the airway
inside the larynx. Sound requires that air move between the cords in
sufficient volume and velocity to vibrate them and thus produce
sound. If the cords are severely damaged, this may not be possible.

Also, if the trachea is severed below the vocal cords, air exhaled
from the lungs exits through the wound, and not enough would
reach the cords to produce vibrations and thus sound (Figure 16).
People who have had trauma to the larynx or have severe lung disease that requires a permanent tracheotomy (hole cut into the tra-

chea just below the larynx) have to plug the tracheotomy hole in order to speak. Otherwise the air escapes through the hole and never passes through the vocal cords. This is a similar situation to the wound described above.

If the vocal cords and the trachea remain intact, noises and speech would be possible—bubbly, wet, raspy, but still speech.

Where Would an Intoxicated Person Have to Be Shot to Put Him in a Coma for Two Days?

Q: My evil villain is going to shoot someone who is blotto drunk and passed out. Not being a professional killer, he shoots the guy and, thinking he must be dead, leaves the scene.

The questions are these: If he was not found for several hours, could he still be alive and yet remain unconscious for a day or two? If so, in what part of his body would he have to be shot?

A: The scenario you lay out could happen. The two-day period of unconsciousness could not be from the alcohol since it is rapidly metabolized (broken down) by the body, and the victim would wake up after a few hours. If he took in enough alcohol to put him out for two days, he would die in short order from the depressive effects of that much ethanol intake.

Gunshot wounds (GSWs) to most of the body would not lead to a two-day coma. A GSW to the head could. The bullet could enter the skull and damage the brain (which would lead to surgery, a long convalescence, and so forth), or it could simply penetrate the scalp and cause a concussion with or without a fracture of the skull bone (cranium). The concussion could cause a period of unconsciousness, disorientation, confusion, and amnesia, or any combination of these as fits your story.

This type of concussive injury could lead to two days of coma or, more likely, a few hours of coma, and then over the next two days the victim could pass from somnolence (sleepiness and difficulty in arousing) to confusion and disorientation, to periods of wakefulness and progressive lucidity, to being fully awake with intact memory, absolutely no memory of the events, or spotty memory. His amnesia could even be retrograde, which means he would have no memory of events prior to his GSW. This retrograde amnesia could extend back for only a few minutes, a few hours, or, in extreme cases, forever.

I think this type of GSW makes the most sense for your scenario and is entirely plausible. Have the bullet either burrow beneath the scalp—in which case the surgeon could remove it under local anesthesia—or bounce off the skull and exit the scalp entirely. When he is found unconscious, he would be taken to the hospital emergency department, where an ER physician and a surgeon would care for him.

X rays would easily determine if the skull was fractured or not, if the bullet entered the brain cavity or not, or if any bullet fragments were left behind within the scalp after the bullet exited. If the bullet did not enter the brain cavity or fracture the skull, the surgeon would remove the bullet and any bullet fragments, clean and dress the wound, and likely place a surgical drain (a short piece of soft rubber tubing) into the wound to allow drainage of body fluids from the injured area. This lessens the incidence of infection. Closing such "dirty wounds" with sutures would allow collection of these bodily fluids within the wound. These fluids make a good culture medium and would promote the growth of infectious bacteria.

The victim would remain in the hospital for several days and receive intravenous antibiotics. At least twice a day the wound would be examined for signs of infection (redness, swelling, pain, pus formation), cleaned, and a fresh dressing applied. After several days the drain would be removed. The concussion would resolve, and the victim would be essentially normal again.

How Did David Kill Goliath?

Q: I have an interesting question for you. It regards the combat between David and Goliath. Other than the Old Testament, there are no historical accounts of which I am aware. I hope you can help me get the medical details of the combat exactly right. Apparently the rock that David slung did not kill Goliath but only stunned him enough to drop him to the ground, allowing the boy time to separate his head from his neck. The tantalizing single detail is that the rock sunk into his forehead (not his temple). The reference is 1 Samuel 17:48–51. What specifically happened to Goliath from just before the stone landed until just after the neck was severed?

A: Great question.

From the description of the brief combat in 1 Samuel, the rock was embedded in Goliath's forehead, and he "fell upon his face to the Earth." A rock to the head can be merely painful or it can kill. Somewhere in between these results, it can cause a concussion, which like a left hook in boxing can stun the recipient or render him unconscious.

Typically, an object such as a rock would cause "blunt force trauma" and not "penetrating trauma," as with a bullet. A blunt force injury to the head may or may not fracture the skull; may or may not cause unconsciousness; may or may not cause bleeding within the brain; and may or may not kill.

A penetrating head wound, by definition, means that the object breached, or penetrated, the skull. This is a more serious injury since the brain itself is traumatized directly by the object. Such penetrating wounds fracture the skull, but they may or may not cause unconsciousness; may or may not cause bleeding into the brain; and may or may not kill.

The rule here is that whatever happens, happens. I once saw a man injured in an industrial accident where a metal disk flew out of a grinding machine and struck him in the forehead. He was knocked out, but only briefly. When he reached the hospital, the disk protruded from his forehead as if some miniature flying saucer had attacked him. On further exam I found that the disk's leading edge had penetrated his skull and embedded in his brain. He was awake, alert, and neurologically normal. A neurosurgeon removed the disk and he did well, with no residual problems. Could he have died instantly? Yes. Could he have bled into his brain and required more extensive surgery or died from this complication? Yes. Could he have suffered permanent brain damage? Yes. The point is that none of these happened. Whatever happens, happens.

Now back to David and Goliath. In 1 Samuel 17: 4 it states that Goliath possessed a height of "six cùbits and a span." Many experts feel that a cubit was roughly 17 inches, while a span was approximately 9 inches, which means Goliath was over 9 feet tall. If this story is true and not merely a parable, Goliath most likely suffered from both gigantism and acromegaly. These conditions are typically caused by tumors of the pituitary gland, which secrete excess amounts of growth hormone (GH). GH causes lengthening and thickening of bones and muscles. Before puberty and the closing of the epiphyses (growth plates) in the bones, persons so affected grow very tall and have long arms and legs. After the epiphyses close, bones no longer can grow lengthwise, but under the continued influence of excess GH, they grow thick. This is particularly true of the hands, feet, jaw, and forehead. Acromegalics have thick hands and fingers, square, shovel-like jaws, and thick, protruding foreheads that seem to cantilever over their eyes. Remember Andre the Giant, the professional wrestler? He is a perfect example. Like Andre, Goliath must have developed a GH-producing pituitary tumor at an early age, and grown very tall, and then in his teens and twenties the continued excess of GH made him muscular and thick-boned.

If Goliath did suffer from acromegaly, it is likely that David's stone embedded in the flesh of the giant's forehead but did not penetrate the skull. In other words, a blunt force injury. Goliath was stunned or rendered unconscious by the concussive blow, and death came when David severed his spinal cord with his sword. In France this type of death was served up by the guillotine.

Of course, if David hurled the stone with enough velocity (with or without the aid of a divine hand), the missile could have penetrated the skull, resulting in a penetrating head wound. Death could have come from this or from the later beheading.

The passages that cover the battle are somewhat confusing. Verse 50 says, "David prevailed over the Philistine with a sling and with a stone, and smote the Philistine, and slew him." Verse 51 says, "David ran and stood upon the Philistine, and took his sword, and drew it out of the sheath thereof, and slew him." Did he slay him with the stone or the sword? Did he merely "prevail" over Goliath with the stone and then slay him with the sword?

I would suspect that David knocked Goliath unconscious, or nearly so, with a blunt force injury from the stone, which embedded in the flesh of Goliath's forehead but did not penetrate his skull, and then David finished him with the beheading. But I could be wrong.

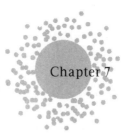

Chapter 7

POISONS AND DRUGS

Is There a Drug or Poison That Mimics Death but Allows the Victim to Survive?

Q: Is there a drug that truly mimics death to the point that a not-so-careful physician might pronounce death and then leave, after which the victim recovers? If so, how would the drug be administered, how long would the effects last, and is there an antidote?

A: You're going to love this. Zombie Powder. Yes, Zombie Powder. It is the toxin of the puffer fish, also called the blowfish. The toxin is called tetraodontoxin or tetradotoxin (I've seen it written as either and also abbreviated as TTX), and it is found in the ovaries of the blowfish. The toxin is not destroyed by cooking, but if the entrails are removed before preparation, the fish itself is harmless.

In Japan the dish is prepared in a manner that leaves a little of the toxin behind. It is called fugu and is a delicacy. The residual toxin, in small doses, gives the diner a flushed and tingly feeling. The fish must be prepared to perfection, or it can be deadly—kind of like gastronomic Russian roulette. The chefs who do this are specially trained and licensed, and even these guys screw up from time to time. Recently, maybe a year or two ago, I read about several deaths in Japan from this.

In Haiti the toxin is used in certain voodoo religious rituals, and it is used in the "zombification" of field-workers and others. It can be sprinkled on the skin of the victim or added to his food, and it takes effect in a few minutes or up to four hours or so. It absorbs through the skin or the gastrointestinal tract.

It is basically a neurotoxin (affects the neurologic system) and causes paralysis, speech difficulty, slow, shallow respirations, and a decreased heart rate, with a weak and thready pulse. The victim may appear dead and is indeed fairly close. The skin of the victim is cool and pale, his breathing slow and shallow, and with an almost unpalpable pulse, one could easily assume the victim was dead.

If he survived the first twenty-four hours, without treatment he would gradually come around over the next two or three days. Proper treatment is directed toward preventing brain damage (see below) and would consist of hospitalization and giving oxygen and drugs to support the blood pressure while the toxin's effects wore off.

How to make a zombie? you ask. Simple. Sprinkle some of the powder in the victim's food or in his shoes. He will become dizzy, short of breath, and weak, and collapse. Then lay him in a shallow ditch, cover him with leaves, and come back in about twelve hours. He will be calm, controllable, and a good field-worker.

What causes this is an anoxic encephalopathy, which means the brain is damaged due to the lack of an adequate oxygen supply. This is the same type of brain injury that occurs in victims of drowning, cardiac arrest, carbon monoxide poisoning, and asphyxiation from any cause. In the case of tetraodontoxin poisoning, the low heart rate and blood pressure and slowed breathing causes the concentration of oxygen in the blood to fall to very low levels, which damages the brain—sort of a metabolic "frontal lobotomy." The surgical version of this happened to Jack Nicholson in *One Flew over the Cookoo's Nest*.

In the 1980s this happened to one of my patients. According to Joe (not his real name, of course), he owned a factory in Haiti, and Jean Claude Duvalier, a.k.a. "Baby Doc," wanted it, but Joe refused to sell. So Baby Doc had some of his Tonton Macoutes goons "zombie-ize" Joe and took his factory. They slipped into his house at night and powdered his shoes. The next thing Joe remembered was waking up three days later, in a three-hundred-year-old prison with rats gnawing on his toes. It took the U.S. State Department a month to get him out of Haiti.

Where would you get this stuff? Haiti, for sure, or perhaps in the Algiers area of New Orleans, where voodoo is still heavily practiced.

What Poison That Can Be Secreted in a Glass Will Kill Instantly When Swallowed?

Q: In my story a poison is placed in a glass. The victim then pours water into the glass and drinks it, dying immediately. At first glance it looks as though he has had a heart attack. However, my sleuth suspects he was poisoned. What poison would fit this scenario, and what clues would tip off my sleuth that the victim was indeed poisoned?

A: There are several possibilities for your scenario, but one excellent choice: cyanide. It is quick, nasty, and effective. Even if someone attempted to save the victim, it is nearly impossible because treatment must begin immediately if any chance of survival is to be realized. Why? Cyanide is a "metabolic poison" in that it basically shuts down the ability of the body's cells to use oxygen. The red blood cells cannot carry oxygen to the tissues, and the tissues of the body can't use the oxygen anyway. It is as if all the oxygen is removed from the body instantly. This process is immediate and profound, and leads to death in one to ten minutes depending on the dosage. So even if CPR is begun immediately, the body cells still can't use the oxygen supplied by this process.

Symptoms are rapid breathing, shortness of breath, dizziness, flushing, nausea, vomiting, loss of consciousness, maybe seizure activity, and then death. These are also common symptoms of a heart attack. This sequence of symptoms happens very quickly, in a matter of seconds or minutes. The victim develops sudden, severe shortness of breath and a flushed face; he may clutch at his chest, collapse to the floor, and die, with or without having a seizure in the process. Also, his skin appears very pink, and if the victim hits his head or scrapes an elbow and bleeds, the blood is a noticeably bright cherry red. This is also true in carbon monoxide poisoning.

Your sleuth could suspect cyanide poisoning from the sudden onset of breathing difficulty followed by a sudden collapse. The pinkish skin color and the bright red color of the victim's blood would be additional clues.

Hydrogen cyanide is a gas and would not fit your situation. It is primarily used in fumigation and can be lethal if inhaled or absorbed through the skin. It is the gas used in gas chamber executions.

Potassium cyanide (KCN) and sodium cyanide (NaCN) are your best bets. They are white powders with a faint bitter almond smell, which most people do not notice. Either could easily be sprinkled into a glass, especially if the glass was opaque, colored, or etched. Both are very powerful and only a small amount would be needed. They readily dissolve in water, alcohol, or a mixed drink.

One caveat: Your killer must be careful when handling KCN or NaCN. They are both easily absorbed through the skin and could do in your killer. Rubber gloves and a complete avoidance of direct contact with the powder would be wise.

KCN and NaCN are used commercially in metal recovery such as extracting gold or silver from their ores and in electroplating such metals as gold, silver, copper, and platinum. They could be pilfered from a jewelry or metal plating company. They are also sold by several chemical supply firms.

In your story a small amount of the powder could be put in the glass and swirled to coat the inside. When the water is added and consumed, the victim would collapse and die very quickly.

Can Ingested Cocaine Kill?

Q: In my story the victim is killed by ingesting cocaine placed in his drink, a Manhattan. The vermouth would probably hide any possible taste. I have read a book on poisons and thought this was feasible. Is it possible? Cyanide would be easier and faster, but for my murderer cocaine was readily available.

A: The short answer is yes, cocaine would work and could work very quickly if the dose is large enough.

Cocaine revs up the brain and can cause seizures, and these can be lethal, especially if they trigger a condition known as status epilepticus. Typically, seizures are self-limited, running their course in a couple of minutes and then ceasing. But in status (for short) they continue sometimes for hours or even days. IV medications such as Dilantin, phenobarbital, or one of the other anticonvulsant (antiseizure) drugs sometimes won't break them. Occasionally, we have to paralyze these types of patients with Anectine (a curare-like drug that paralyzes all muscles—not just the seizing ones but also those needed for respiration) and place them on a ventilator until things settle down. This prevents them from dying from lack of ventilation or aspiration of stomach contents. Breaking these types of seizures can take several days in severe situations.

Even without status a seizure can be lethal since it interferes with respiration or can lead to vomiting and aspiration. More likely, however, the cocaine would cause some cardiac event such as the following:

1. *Lethal cardiac arrhythmias* (irregularity in the heart's normal rhythm): Ventricular tachycardia or ventricular fibrillation may occur as a result of the direct effect of cocaine's stimulat-

ing properties. Most people who die suddenly after cocaine use do so from this type of change in the cardiac rhythm. It may occur after ingestion, snorting, intravenous (IV) injection, or freebasing, which is the smoking of cocaine. With freebasing the cocaine is absorbed through the lungs almost as fast as if given by IV.

2. *Coronary arterial spasm* (narrowing from the contraction of the muscles in the walls of the arteries): The coronary arteries are the ones that supply blood to the heart muscle. When they spasm, the flow of blood can be severely and even completely restricted, and the area of the heart supplied by that artery may die (heart attack, myocardial infarction, or MI) or a lethal arrhythmia, as described above, may result secondary to poor blood flow to the heart muscle. This is not uncommon, and I have seen several patients over the years with this occurrence.

Crack cocaine, because of its greater concentration and delivery through the lungs, is particularly dangerous.

In your scenario the ingestion of cocaine from a spiked drink could cause all the above. A seizure, a heart attack, or a sudden death from an arrhythmia or any combination could happen. The victim may clutch his chest and complain of shortness of breath, become pale, and sweat profusely—exactly like a heart attack. He may fall to the floor in a grand mal seizure. His back would arch, his eyes roll back, and powerful jerking motions of his arms and legs would occur. He might bite his tongue, causing it to bleed, or he might vomit and aspirate. In the case of the arrhythmia, the victim would simply collapse and die. Fade to black, cut, print, roll the credits.

One more thought: Cocaine is bitter and is a local anesthetic that numbs the victim's mouth. However, the taste can be masked, especially if it is the victim's third or fourth drink. And since the absorption rate of cocaine by the GI tract is fairly rapid by the time the victim senses the numbing effect or otherwise figures out that something is amiss, he might be on the floor with no pulse. Additionally, if the victim is not a user, his tolerance for an acute dose of cocaine is greatly reduced so that a smaller dose can prove lethal.

What Happens in Carbon Monoxide Poisoning?

Q: I am working on a story in which one of the characters is murdered by piping the exhaust from a gasoline engine into the room where she is sleeping. What actually happens in this circumstance? What causes death? I read that people who die in this manner have bright red skin. True? Why? How long after she lost consciousness would she still have a chance to survive if found?

A: The culprit in exposure to exhaust from a gas-powered engine is carbon monoxide (CO). It can also come from a faulty gas heater or a fireplace where the gas or the wood are incompletely burned. Complete combustion of gas or wood forms carbon dioxide (CO_2), the same gas we exhale with each breath. Though high levels of CO_2 can be harmful and even deadly (this is what happens when people suffocate in car trunks, abandoned refrigerators, vaults, and so forth), CO_2 is not nearly as toxic as CO.

Our red blood cells (RBCs) contain hemoglobin, which is an iron-containing molecule that binds oxygen and carries it to our tissues, where it is released. The tissue cells then use the oxygen for all their vital processes. Inhaled CO is rapidly absorbed through the lungs and into the bloodstream, where it binds with hemoglobin with an affinity 210 times that of oxygen. This means that if air is inhaled that contains CO, the hemoglobin prefers to take on the CO and not the oxygen. The cells can't use CO, so the net effect is that they are suffocated.

The combining of CO with hemoglobin produces carboxyhemoglobin, which gives the blood a bright cherry red color. It is true that people dying from CO poisoning can have a bright red color to their skin and the mucous membranes inside the mouth, but not always. Cyanosis causes the skin to have a blue-gray color and it occurs due to lack of oxygen; this duskiness may mask the red hue from the carboxyhemoglobin.

Most fatal cases are found to have carboxyhemoglobin levels in their blood of 50 percent or more, though the old, young, and chronically ill may succumb to levels as low as 25 to 30 percent. This is particularly true of people with chronic heart or lung disease.

At autopsy the M.E. would suspect CO poisoning from the history (the victim being found in a garage with a car engine running), the reddish color of the internal tissues, and the cherry red hue of the blood. This cherry red color of the blood usually requires a concentration of carboxyhemoglobin greater than 30 percent. The skin in dependent areas, where the blood settles after death, are most likely to show the characteristic red color, but this may be masked by the purplish blue color of the dependent lividity. Even in these situations, however, the margins of the lividity may show the red color. The M.E. would then test the blood for carboxyhemoglobin in order to determine if it was the cause of death.

By the time she absorbed enough CO to lose consciousness, she would be very near the point where she would suffer permanent brain damage and death.

As to how long your victim could survive after losing consciousness, there is no exact answer since too many variables are involved. Her age, weight, and general health status; the concentration of the CO; how airtight the room was; and what drugs or alcohol, if any, she consumed prior to exposure are just a few of the things to consider. A ballpark would be half an hour at the outside; fifteen minutes would be better. If you need to make it an hour or so, provide some sort of ventilation into the garage—something the killer didn't notice that would supply just enough fresh air to extend the time of death a little. It might be an open window, or perhaps the family dog comes to investigate after the bad guys leave and pushes open the door that leads from the house to the garage, thus allowing some fresh air to enter.

What Duration of Exposure to Natural Gas Would Be Required to Kill a Person?

Q: I'm setting up an attempted murder. A character goes home, gets roaring drunk, and passes out. Then somebody sneaks into his house, turns on the gas stove, and blows out the pilot light. Any idea on how long it would take the guy to die or, in this case, how long he can be in there without dying? I want him to get sick but survive with no ill effects.

A: This is a difficult if not impossible question to answer, which is a good thing for story crafting. There are lots of options.

The effect of the gas on the person depends on three things in general: the concentration of the gas inhaled, the duration of exposure, and the condition of the victim prior to the event.

The concentration would depend on the flow from the gas jet, the size of the room or house, and the amount and character of ventilation in the room. A small studio apartment would fill with gas more quickly than a 5,000-square-foot house. Also, the victim would likely be closer to the point of origin of the gas. A studio would have the kitchen area and the sleeping area in the same room, as opposed to the bedroom being down the hall or upstairs from the kitchen in a house. Open windows, ceiling fans, or the air-conditioning system would supply some degree of ventilation and prolong the intended victim's survival. Of course, the electrical circuits of the fan or air conditioning could trigger an explosion once the gas concentration reached a certain level, but that doesn't fit your scenario.

The exposure time is self-explanatory. The longer the exposure at any given gas concentration, the more likely death would occur.

The condition of the victim plays a role because people with heart or lung disease, diabetes, liver or kidney problems, and certain other medical conditions would be more susceptible than the average person. Also, alcohol or other sedative drugs would interfere with the cough reflex and impair the victim's ability to recognize the symptoms of exposure (cough, shortness of breath, headache, an unpleasant taste in the mouth, blurred vision, and so forth), thus lessening the likelihood that he would realize what was happening until it was too late.

Why is this confusion good? Because you have great leeway in how you handle the plot. Whether it's an hour or several hours and whether your victim survives or not is up to you. I wouldn't leave him in the room overnight or all day, particularly if his home is a small apartment. Most people would die from even moderate levels of exposure for that amount of time. Otherwise, make it fit what you want.

What Substance Could Be Added to Water to Hasten Death in Someone Stranded in a Desert?

Q: In my story a young man is released deep in the desert with only a bottle of water. Is there a substance that could be added to the water that would hasten dehydration and death?

A: Two very simple ones: alcohol and diuretics.

Alcohol acts like a diuretic, as anyone who has had a couple of beers knows. Remember, you don't buy beer, you merely rent it. Alcohol depresses the posterior lobe of the pituitary gland, which makes a hormone called antidiuretic hormone (ADH). This hormone causes the kidneys to hold on to water. The depressing effect of alcohol decreases the amount of ADH released and thus what reaches the kidneys. The result is that the kidneys "open up," and urine volume increases dramatically. Thus, alcohol is a diuretic.

Diuretics are a class of drugs that, by several different mechanisms, force the kidneys to filter more water from the bloodstream and produce more urine. Common ones are hydrochlorothiazide (HCTZ), Dyazide, and Lasix (furosemide). HCTZ and Dyazide are mild, while Lasix is powerful. In fact, a single dose of Lasix may bring about the loss of several quarts of water. That is why this particular medication is useful and at times lifesaving for the treatment of individuals with heart failure and pulmonary edema, a condition in which the body is severely fluid overloaded and the lungs are filled with water.

In your situation you could dissolve a 40-milligram Lasix tablet in the water. It has little taste, but to make sure no funny taste is detected, Gatorade or fruit juice could be used. In this case the killer would give the victim a liquid that the victim believes is lifesaving, while in reality the concoction will only make things much worse. Depending on the temperature, the terrain the victim must cross, the dryness of the air, and the size, age, and health of the victim, it may take a couple of days for him to reach a life-threatening level of dehydration. The addition of Lasix to his water supply may cut this to a few hours.

Is There a Drug That Not Only Subdues a Victim but Also Erases Her Memory?

Q: Situation: A woman pulls into her garage, opens her car door, and is attacked by someone who wants her temporarily unconscious. Can he give her a rap in that magical spot under the jaw or thereabouts and momentarily knock her out? Would that blot out her immediately previous memory? Or could he give her a jab in the arm with some quick-acting drug that would work for a while, so that she comes to in a hour or so and is not permanently damaged?

A: Yes, you can knock someone out with a blow to the head, jaw, temple, and even the neck. It requires the blow to be delivered with enough force to disrupt brain function and thus cause a loss of consciousness. This is a "concussion" in medical terms. Usually the victim wakes up in a minute or two, but she could be out longer. Fifteen minutes or a half hour—either is possible.

In the movies the hero knocks someone out with one punch, but in real life it is not always that easy and may require several blows. The hero then forgets about the unconscious henchman, as if he were suddenly written out of the script, and continues to pursue the main villain. How many times have you seen that? The truth is that the henchman is likely to awaken in a couple of minutes, get himself together, and surprise the hero, who was sure he would never be a problem again. At least that is the way the script reads. Another case of art *not* imitating life.

In your situation, if the villain needs her out for only a few minutes to a half hour, a single blow to the back of the head is realistic. If he needs her unconscious for an hour or more, the blow to the head isn't enough.

The problem with memory loss is that it is unpredictable. Sometimes it occurs, sometimes it doesn't. What you are proposing is "retrograde amnesia," which is a backward loss of memory—that is, the loss of memory for events that occurred prior to the injury. This is even less likely but certainly does happen. Victims of major auto accidents who are knocked out may not remember leaving home in the car or where they were going.

Your victim could be surprised and never really see the attacker. Then memory is not part of the equation. Or you could have her see the attacker and suffer retrograde amnesia. In the latter case the memory may return later. This is a good plot twist and something for the assailant to worry about.

Drugs are a more difficult problem since few drugs act instantly. Some act in a few seconds, but to do so they must be given intravenously. A drug such as sodium pentothal would fit this situation.

Your victim could be overpowered and an IV injection given, but this would probably require two attackers since it's hard to hold someone down and find a vein with a needle at the same time. Another route that is almost as fast as an IV is an injection under, in, or around the tongue. The tongue is so highly vascular that it's almost like giving the drug intravenously. That's why nitroglycerin is taken under the tongue by patients with angina and why many drug addicts use this area when their veins are scarred beyond use.

Another possible scenario for you might be for the attacker to approach from behind and knock out or stun the victim with a blow to the back of the head. He then can give a drug that makes her compliant and blocks her memory. Maybe he needs her help to find whatever he is after in her house or something like that.

The perfect drug for this would be Versed (midazolam), manufactured by Roche Pharmaceuticals. It can be given intravenously in a dose of 2 to 4 milligrams (mg) or intramuscularly in a dose of 5 to 10 mg. It works within a minute and has a sedative effect. More important, it causes almost complete amnesia for its duration of action, which is two to five hours. The victim would be very pliable, would follow commands, could walk and talk, and may appear normal or slightly sedated but would have absolutely no memory of what happens. Your attacker could knock out your victim with a blow to the head and then inject about 5 mg of Versed in her arm or hip, and when the victim wakes up from the blow a few minutes later she would be under the influence of the drug and remember nothing of what happens over the following several hours. This might work well for you.

Is There a Toxic Pesticide That Can Be Disseminated by Fire or an Explosion?

Q: In my novel a ship loaded with a pesticide banned by the Food and Drug Administration for its toxic effects docks in a harbor. The ship is sabotaged with incendiary devices and catches fire. The pesticide tanks rupture, producing a toxic gas that sickens and kills people in the harbor. Is this possible? If so, what pesticide could be on board?

A: There are several that fit your scenario.

Sarin and parathion are anticholinesterase neurotoxins. They block the cholinesterase enzymes that are necessary for proper functioning of the muscles and nerves. It is complicated physiology that would take literally thousands of words to explain. Fortunately, you don't really need to know the details to write a credible scene.

Parathion is a yellowish brown liquid that is used as an insecticide and to kill ascaria worms. It also comes as a gas that is quickly absorbed through the skin or lungs. The victim dies a horrible death. Symptoms begin in thirty to sixty minutes and include constricted (small) pupils, muscle spasms and weakness, involuntary twitching, nausea, vomiting, diarrhea, cardiac arrhythmias, a burning sensation in the skin, and pulmonary edema (lungs filled with water). Respiratory failure and death soon follow.

Sarin is even more toxic. A single drop on the skin can be deadly. It doesn't damage the skin but quickly penetrates it and enters the bloodstream. It is particularly dangerous if heated or if mixed with water or steam because it releases extremely toxic fumes.

An explosion and fire on the ship that ruptured or burned the tanks carrying these compounds would be a disaster of the first order. Injury and death would occur throughout the harbor. Treatment of victims is difficult and not very successful,

Another possibility would be Dieldrin. It is banned in the United States since the 1974 Environmental Protection Agency Act, but it is manufactured in Europe. A white crystalline solid that comes as a spray, powder, or dust, it absorbs through the skin or lungs. When it is heated, it releases an extremely toxic chloride gas. Symptoms, which can begin in twenty minutes, include headache, dizziness, nausea, vomiting, sweating, seizures, and death. As with sarin and parathion, treatment is symptomatic and marginally beneficial.

Any of these would fit your needs and would produce widespread and dramatic injuries and death.

Are Some Poisons Absorbed Through the Skin?

Q: Is it true that your skin absorbs some poisons? If so, what are some common ones?

A: The skin is our largest organ. More than simply a "jacket to keep everything inside," it is a living entity that is affected by many things, both internal and external. Many internal diseases manifest changes in the skin, as do things that contact it from the outside. Sunburn, bumps, bruises, scrapes, and irritative chemicals are some common ones.

Yes, chemical substances, including some medicines and poisons, are absorbed through the skin. Many medicines are now available in transdermal delivery systems. Adhesive patches can deliver nicotine for smoking cessation, nitroglycerin for angina, clonidine for hypertension, and scopolamine for motion sickness, just to name a few.

Heavy metals such as antimony, mercury, and lead pass through the skin and can result in chronic poisoning. DDT, chlordane, paraquat, malathion, and other pesticides cross the skin barrier and can cause acute and chronic problems. Cyanide readily slips through and can be very deadly.

An interesting historical note is that Ludwig van Beethoven may have died from plumbism (lead poisoning). Recently evaluated samples of his hair contained one hundred times the normal level of lead. His exposure could have come from pewter dishes and drinking vessels, leaded paint, or perhaps from water pipes, which contained lead in his day. However, another source could have been a glass harmonica. This instrument, which produced a hypnotic wet crystal sound, was invented by Benjamin Franklin in 1761. He demonstrated the instrument to Beethoven and Wolfgang Amadeus Mozart on his visit to France during the American Revolutionary War. Both composers later wrote music for the instrument.

The glass harmonica consisted of various-sized blown glass bowls arrayed along a spindle that rotated while the player placed moistened fingers on the bowls. Leaded paint was applied to the bowls to differentiate the various notes each would produce. Perhaps the lead that invaded Beethoven's body entered through his fingers or from licking them to keep them moist, which was necessary to produce the sounds.

The symptoms of chronic plumbism include psychiatric and neurologic problems, deafness, and eventually death. It sounds a lot like Ludwig. Wolfgang, too, for that matter.

Does Jimsonweed Make an Effective Poison?

Q: Can an adult die from drinking a strong tea made with jimsonweed?

A: Jimsonweed *(Datura stramonium)* is also called devil's trumpet, stinkweed, and thorn apple. It typically grows in warmer climates. It was originally called Jamestown weed because soldiers sent to fight Bacon's Rebellion in 1666 in Jamestown, Virginia, ran out of food and ate the berries of this plant, resulting in a mass poisoning.

The plant has white or purple funnel-shaped flowers and possesses an unpleasant odor. It also has a very unpleasant taste, so tea may not work. Perhaps you might consider a more aromatic drink such as mulled cider or a Manhattan (it contains vermouth and bitters, which might mask the taste, particularly if it was the victim's third or fourth drink).

The entire plant is poisonous, and when burned, the fumes are toxic. A tea made from the leaves and/or seeds is particularly toxic. In your scenario you could boil several of the plants in a pot of water until a strong liquor remained. Add this to any drink, and it would be very toxic.

The poisonous ingredients are hyoscyamine (mostly), hyoscine, and atropine. They are in the belladonna alkaloid family, with the prototype being the belladonna plant, or deadly nightshade, as it is also called.

Death may take several hours, depending on the strength of the tea and the amount ingested. Symptoms are those of atropine poisoning: vertigo, blurred vision, dilated pupils, headache, rapid and weak pulse, drowsiness, mania, delirium, confusion, disorientation, dry mouth and eyes, extreme thirst, flushing and a burning sensation of the skin, seizures, and finally coma and death.

In medical school we learned the signs and symptoms of atropine poisoning as follows:

> Blind as a bat (dilated pupils and blurred vision)
> Red as a beet (the skin may become red and burn)
> Dry as a bone (the dry eyes and mouth)
> Mad as a hatter (the mania and delirium)

As you see, you have numerous symptoms and signs to work with. These can occur in almost any combination, since people react differently to the toxins.

How Does the "Posture" of Strychnine Poisoning Work?

Q: I am writing a mystery where the murdered character has been given a lethal dose of strychnine via eyedrops and dumped in a field where he dies. He is then buried by the killer. The body is found approximately three weeks later. I have read that strychnine poisoning causes a classic death grin on the face of a victim, blue coloring of the skin, and bowing of the back muscles, which is evident on a corpse after death. Am I correct about this? I want my victim to reflect the obvious postmortem symptoms of strychnine poisoning so that when the body is discovered, the M.E. recognizes these conditions and suspects strychnine as the cause of death. Is waiting three weeks for discovery of the body too long for this to be feasible? How about the use of eyedrops to administer strychnine? What's the average time and dosage for it to take effect and start seizures?

A: First, let's look at strychnine. It comes from several types of plants and their seeds. One source is the dog button *(Strychnos nux-vomica),* which grows in tropical areas, such as India and Hawaii. It is a colorless, odorless crystalline powder with a bitter taste. It can absorb through the stomach, the lungs, the skin, and the conjunctivae (the pink part) of the eyes.

The problem with your chosen method of delivery of this poison is one of dosing. The lethal amount of strychnine is between 100 and 120 milligrams (mg), and it would be difficult to concentrate the powder sufficiently so that a couple of drops in the eye would be lethal. Perhaps you could put it in the saline solution the victim uses to wash his eyes if he is a contact lens wearer. This would be more plausible since irrigating his eyes with the tainted solution after removing his contacts might supply enough of the drug to do him in. A more realistic choice would be to add it to food or drink, but I do like the idea of introducing the poison through the eyes. It's a good twist.

Strychnine works in ten to twenty minutes, and its effects are very dramatic. It is a neurologic toxin that attacks the central nervous system and typically causes seizurelike muscular activity before death. It does not cause true grand mal seizures, which result from chaotic electrical impulses in the brain. Rather, strychnine attacks the nerves that enervate the muscles.

Symptoms begin with the victim's developing a stiffness in his neck and face, followed by spasms in his arms and legs. Any sound or movement can trigger a wave of erratic and powerful muscular contractions. These spastic contractions increase, and the large muscles of the back begin to contract, pulling the body into an arched position (a posture called opisthotonus). These symptoms are similar to those found in tetanus. The victim dies of asphyxia since he cannot breathe.

At death the victim usually has an arched back, eyes wide open, and the mouth pulled into a broad grimace—called the death smile, or *risus sardonicus.* This is the stuff of nightmares.

Rigor mortis typically sets in immediately in deaths associated with violent muscular activity, as is seen in strychnine poisonings, so that the body is frozen in this posture. The reason that rigor occurs quickly is that the violent contractions of the muscles consume the intramuscular enzymes (predominately adenosine triphosphate, or ATP). In typical rigor mortis it is the depletion of these enzymes that causes the muscles to contract, producing the rigid phase of rigor. In situations such as strychnine poisoning or deaths associated with seizure activity, this depletion of the ATP occurs more rapidly, so that the rigid phase of rigor occurs more quickly. Over the next twenty-four hours, as the muscles decompose, they lose their contractile property, causing the relaxation phase of rigor.

Your victim will thus have a very quick onset of the rigid phase and will hold this strychnine posture—arched back, grimacing smile, eyes wide—for twelve to twenty-four hours or so. Then, as the rigor resolves, the muscles will relax, and the face and body will, too. So three weeks won't work. He would look like any other three-week-old corpse, and the M.E. would have to perform toxicologic tests to determine the presence of strychnine.

What Is the Lethal Dose of Strychnine in Humans and in Various Animals?

Q: I have a question about strychnine as a poison. What dosages would kill a mouse, a rat, a cat, a dog, a monkey, and then a human? My criminal is going to do some experiments that will ultimately lead to his poisoning his victim.

A: The lethal dose in the average adult human is 100 to 120 milligrams (mg). The average adult weighs 70 kilograms (kg), or about 154 pounds (1 kg equals 2.2 lb). That calculates to a lethal dose of 1.4 to 1.7 mg per kg, or 0.65 to 0.78 mg per lb. So if we take an average lethal dose of 0.7 mg per pound, we can estimate the following lethal doses:

2 oz (⅛ lb) mouse	0.09 mg
1 lb rat	0.70 mg
8 lb cat	5.60 mg
15 lb dog	10.50 mg
25 lb monkey	17.50 mg
180 lb man	126 mg

This assumes that strychnine works in these various mammalian species in the same way, which it probably does. Regardless, these should be ballpark numbers.

Is There a Poison That Causes Stomach Distention and Death?

Q: For a short story I'm writing I'd like the victim, who is pregnant, to die with a distended stomach. Whatever poison I use has to be put into a drink. Could lead poisoning lead to a quick death? I've read that the effect is slow and progressive. What would be the effect on the fetus? And what would be the best source of lead that could be camouflaged in a drink?

A: Lead can be used as an acute poison, but it is more of a cumulative poison. Chronic exposure causes a multitude of medical problems and ultimately death. A large dose taken orally could do the trick but would be difficult to hide in a drink. Toxic forms would be lead carbonate, lead monoxide, and lead sulfate. The most toxic would be lead arsenate because it contains arsenic. It is a white powder and is found in many pesticides and veterinary tapeworm medicine. This could be dissolved in a drink and would do the trick. For that matter, arsenic would, too. A popular poison for centuries, it has become a cliché, as you know, but it works.

Acute arsenic poisoning causes a breakdown of the lining of the stomach and intestines with bleeding. It inflames the blood vessels and causes them to leak. This leads to gastrointestinal (GI) bleeding and pulmonary edema, which is the accumulation of fluid in the lungs. Also, vomiting, abdominal pain, and diarrhea, sometimes bloody, can occur. Finally, delirium, seizures, coma, and death occur.

Another choice might be mercury. Found in thermometers and

some batteries, it is readily available. It is more potent if the vapors are inhaled rather than if it is ingested. It has a low boiling point of about 40 degrees centigrade and 104 degrees Fahrenheit. (Water boils at 100 degrees C. and 212 degrees F.)

Water containing mercury could be boiled. The vapors would enter the air, and the victim would inhale them and die fairly quickly. Symptoms would be nausea, vomiting, abdominal pain, salivation, fever, cough, shortness of breath, and a metallic taste in the mouth. The reaction time is almost immediate. With ingestion the reaction time is about a half hour, and symptoms are similar.

Another very good choice that could fit your scenario is carbon tetrachloride (carbon tet for short). It is found in dry cleaning agents, household spot removers, and some fire extinguishers. Its effects are increased when taken with alcohol. This colorless liquid has a distinctive and strong odor that must be masked. Symptoms are abdominal pain, nausea, vomiting, dizziness, confusion, shortness of breath, shock, coma, and death. It also has a low boiling point, and so a vapor as described above could be produced and would be immediately toxic. Its boiling point is 77 degrees C. and 171 degrees F.

Any of these could also be toxic for the fetus, and, of course, if the victim died, the fetus would, too, unless an emergency cesarean section was performed.

Although any of these would work, I think mercury or carbon tet would be best. I particularly like the idea of a vapor, but that doesn't fit your original plot idea.

How Deadly Are Death Cap Mushrooms, and What Do They Do to the Victim?

Q: In my story a murder is committed by feeding the victim a death cap mushroom. I need to know how quickly it acts and what reactions the victim would have before death.

A: The death cap mushroom *(Amanita phalloides)* is the most dangerous of the mushrooms. In fact, the entire Amanita family is to be avoided. Other toxic species are the fool's mushroom *(A. verna),* the death angel *(A. virosa),* and the smaller death angel *(A. bisporiger).*

The death cap grows in the southeast United States and prefers damp forested areas. The others prefer dry pine forests or mixed wooded areas and lawns. Their cap colors vary from pale green to yellow-olive in the coastal United States and Europe and to white or light brown in the remainder of the United States. All have white gills with white spores on the underside of their caps.

The death cap is so toxic that a single mushroom can kill. The two main toxins found in these mushrooms are amanitin, which causes a drop in blood sugar (hypoglycemia), and phalloidin, which damages the kidneys, liver, and heart. Symptoms are slow in onset, typically beginning six to fifteen hours after ingestion, and they may be delayed as much as forty-eight hours. In general, the later the onset of symptoms, the worse the chances for survival. This is because the toxins go to work on the liver and other organs almost immediately, but the late onset of symptoms delays the seeking of medical help.

Symptoms usually begin with stomach pain, nausea, vomiting, and bloody diarrhea. When the liver is involved, jaundice will impart a yellow hue to the skin. The victim may then lapse into a coma. As the kidneys fail and as dehydration progresses due to vomiting and diarrhea, the potassium level in the blood can rise abruptly and lead to cardiac arrest and death.

Treatment is often not helpful because, as stated above, by the time help is sought, the toxins are already working their mischief in the body. Regardless, the first order of business is to pump the stomach to remove any residual mushrooms. This would help only in the first four to six hours. After that, the mushrooms have been digested and are no longer in the stomach. The victim is monitored with blood tests for hypoglycemia, elevated potassium, and abnormal liver and kidney function. These problems are treated as they arise. Otherwise, hope and prayer are suggested.

A quicker-acting toxin is the panther mushroom *(A. pantherina)* or the fly agaric mushroom *(A. muscaria)*, both members of the Amanita family. They come in a variety of colors, from yellow to red to orange to grayish brown, and often have white patches on their caps. These contain several different poisons. Choline and muscarine cause a drop in blood pressure and pulse, nausea, dizziness, profuse sweating and salivation, tearing of the eyes, and diarrhea. Ibotenic acid and muscimol cause dizziness, headache, seizures, blurred vision, muscle cramping, loss of balance, coma, respiratory failure, and death.

The symptoms typically begin from half an hour to three hours after ingestion. Treatment is similar to the above measures plus the use of atropine to block the effects of the muscarine and choline. Atropine must be given intravenously. Typically, 0.5 to 1 milligram is given every hour as needed to keep the heart rate and blood pressure within normal ranges.

What Drug Available in the Nineteenth Century Could Be Used to Make a Victim Pliant but Awake?

Q: In my story, my protagonist needs to transport a captive by rail in 1889 Europe. What drug would keep the victim semi-mobile but helpless over a weeklong railway trip?

A: I think your best bet would be one of the opium derivatives. Laudanum (tincture of opium) and morphine were widely available. In fact, during the last half of the nineteenth century, laudanum, opium, and morphine were the drugs used most often for suicide in England. These drugs were commonly used for pain, sedation, and to calm crying babies. They weren't controlled substances as they are today. It wasn't until 1909 that an international commission took the first steps toward regulating opium.

Laudanum was probably first created by the great physician Paracelsus. It was the addiction of Samuel Taylor Coleridge (1772–1834) and Sir Walter Scott (1771–1832), who used it to relieve his long-standing abdominal pain from what was likely chronic gallbladder disease.

Opium is a white powder, while the tincture is a liquid. Either could be added to food or drink. The victim would be sleepy, lethargic, and manageable, and the dose could be easily adjusted to give the desired effect. When the victim begins to "lighten up," another dose could be given. The villain could pass off the victim's symptoms as illness rather than drugs, and no one would probably be the wiser. And when the drug is stopped, the victim would return to normal and would likely have only a fuzzy memory of events.

What Were Some Common Poisons Available in Medieval Europe?

Q: What would be some common poisons available to my medieval poisoner? What are their effects?

A: There were many very effective poisons available during the medieval period and before. These are the common ones:

Arsenic: Arsenic is a metal that is grayish in color in its pure form. Most often it is found as arsenic trioxide, which is a white powder. It can easily be added to food, where it is unlikely to be detected.

This was the favorite poison of the treacherous French queen Catherine de Médicis. She also apparently used *aqua toffana* or *aquetta di Napoli*, which was a mixture of arsenic and cantharidin.

Another interesting use of arsenic was in *venin de crapaud*. Arsenic was fed to toads or other small animals, and after they died, the carcasses were cooked to produce juices. These were added to the food or drink of the victim, with extremely toxic results.

Acute poisoning causes severe gastric burning, nausea, vomiting, and bloody diarrhea. The victim's blood pressure drops, and he becomes weak, dizzy, cold, clammy, and confused, and may develop seizures. Death follows these painful and dramatic events.

Belladonna (Atropa belladonna): This is a plant, and it is also called deadly nightshade. One of the active chemicals in belladonna is atropine. The name "atropine" comes from one of the three Greek Fates, Atropos, who wielded the shears that cut the thread of human life. Other active compounds include scopolamine, hyoscyamine, and hyoscine.

One effect of belladonna is to dilate the pupils, and it is from this that its name arose. Women would use a drop in each eye to dilate their pupils, which was thought to enhance their beauty. "Belladonna" means beautiful woman.

All parts of the plant are toxic when swallowed, and symptoms begin within an hour or so of ingestion. The signs and symptoms of atropine poisoning include dilated pupils, blurred vision, dry mouth and eyes, fever, flushed skin, abdominal cramping, confusion, disorientation, seizures, and cardiac arrest.

Cantharidin (Cantharis vericatoria): Also called Spanish fly, it is a tasteless white powder that can be easily secreted in food or drink. Symptoms appear immediately after ingestion. Cantharidin is very irritative to every tissue it contacts, and when it is filtered from the bloodstream by the kidneys, it causes irritation of the urinary tract and thus was felt to be an aphrodisiac. In larger doses it can cause severe burning and blistering of the gastrointestinal and urinary tracts, and lead to abdominal pain, nausea, vomiting of blood, bloody diarrhea, painful and bloody urination, convulsions, a rapid pulse, a drop in blood pressure, shock, and death.

Foxglove (Digitalis purpurea): A beautiful flowering plant it is also called the fairy cap, fairy bells, and fairy thimbles. These plants are the natural source of digitalis, a medication that has been in use for over a century in the treatment of heart failure and certain cardiac arrhythmias.

All parts of the plant are toxic. Symptoms of poisoning begin in a half hour or so. The victim experiences headache, nausea, vomiting, muscle cramping, shortness of breath, dizziness, palpitations, and finally death from cardiac arrest.

Hemlock (Conium maculatum): This is the poison that reputedly killed Socrates. All parts of the plant are poisonous, particularly the fruit during flowering season. The active toxin is coniine, which is a neurotoxin that paralyzes muscles much like curare. Symptoms begin in a half hour, but death may take several hours.

The first symptom is typically a loss of muscular strength, which progresses. Muscle pain and paralysis follow until the respiratory muscles fail and death ensues from asphyxia.

Henbane (Hyoscamus niger): This is also called insane root, fetid nightshade, and poison tobacco. All parts of the plant contain hyoscyamine, a chemical also found in belladonna, and thus the signs and symptoms of poisoning with henbane are similar to those of atropine toxicity. The onset of symptoms occurs in approximately fifteen minutes.

Poisonous mushrooms were also widely available.

What Are the Effects of Rhubarb Ingestion?

Q: One of my characters is fed raw rhubarb leaves torn up in a salad as an attempt to poison her. How soon would she react, and what would the reaction be? If she is taken to the hospital, what treatment would she receive? Are there any long-term complications? What is the recovery period?

A: Rhubarb *(Rheum rhaponticum)* contains oxalic acid, which is the toxic substance in poisonings. It is found in the leaves and also in the stalks of several subspecies of rhubarb. Oxalic acid causes problems in two ways. The first is topical injury due to its irritant effects, and the second is "internal," occurring after it is absorbed into the body.

Oxalic acid is very irritating to the GI tract and causes mouth, throat, and esophageal pain as well as weakness, shortness of breath, stomach pain with nausea, vomiting, and possibly bleeding. Because there is a delayed onset of symptoms, your victim may not know something was wrong for several hours after eating the leaves. This delay is part of what makes rhubarb so treacherous. If it caused vomiting to occur more quickly, less internal damage would result, since the vomiting would empty the stomach. The amount of the oxalic acid that gets absorbed is directly related to how long the rhubarb remains in the stomach. Less time, less absorption, less internal problems.

These internal problems are due to the chemical properties of oxalic acid. When oxalic acid is absorbed into the bloodstream, it reacts with calcium in the blood to form calcium oxalate. This reaction consumes the blood's calcium, and the level of calcium falls to low levels. Since calcium is necessary for the proper electrical function of the heart, these low levels can cause cardiac arrest and death. Also, the calcium oxalate produced in the bloodstream by this chemical reaction is filtered through the kidneys, where it can clog up the microscopic tubules and severely damage the kidneys. This can cause burning urination and lead to permanent loss of kidney function. Dialysis and/or kidney transplantation may be required.

The first steps in treatment consist of emptying any residual plant from the stomach and neutralizing any oxalic acid to prevent its absorption. The more quickly this is done, the better. Forced vomiting, using an emetic (a drug that causes vomiting), or stomach lavage (washing out the stomach with a tube inserted through the nose and into the stomach) will remove any residual plant product. A common emetic is ipecac syrup. A couple of teaspoons given orally will cause vomiting in five to ten minutes. Then milk or any other calcium-containing liquid can be given orally or via the lavage tube. This binds up, or reacts with, the oxalate before it gets absorbed. In this way the calcium oxalate is formed in the stomach rather than in the bloodstream, where it works its worst mischief, and can be lavaged away.

Also, calcium in the form of calcium gluconate is given by a slow intravenous (IV) drip to raise the calcium level in the blood to normal. Large amounts of IV fluids are given to flush the kidneys and remove any oxalate before it can damage them.

In the emergency room your victim would likely have a thick rubber lavage tube passed through her nose and into her stomach. The stomach would be lavaged with milk or calcium citrate. An IV would be placed for calcium gluconate infusion and to give several liters of D5NS (5 percent dextrose normal saline solution), and blood tests would be run to evaluate kidney function and assess blood calcium levels. An EKG would be done immediately, and she would be admitted to the ICU for monitoring of her cardiac rhythm.

Prognosis and long-term problems would depend on the degree of exposure and the rapidity of treatment. Recovery could be as short as twenty-four hours if treatment is effective and no cardiac or kidney complications occur, and she could have no long-term problems. Or she could suffer cardiac arrest and undergo CPR. She could suffer kidney failure and require short- or long-term dialysis, or she may need a kidney transplant at a later date.

Does Selenium Make an Effective Poison?

Q: I read recently about a murder case involving selenium and might want to use this in my current novel. What is selenium, and how does it work as a poison? What are the symptoms of poisoning, and if the intended victim survived, what medical treatment would be required?

A: Selenium is a nonmetallic element in the same chemical family as sulfur, oxygen, polonium, and tellurium. It is an essential element for life, and its deficiency can lead to various medical problems, the most important being cardiomyopathy (a weakening of the heart muscle). Interestingly, Marco Polo may have discovered the first cases of selenium poisoning when he described a disease called "hoof rot," which occurred in horses in the Nan Shan and Tien Shan Mountains of Turkestan. The soil in that area is rich in selenium.

Selenium poisoning is rare, although it does occur in industrial situations. Its principal applications are in the manufacture of glass, ceramics, photoelectric cells, semiconductors, steel, and vulcanized rubber. The most toxic forms are selenium dioxide (SeO_2) and selenious acid (H_2SeO_4).

Acute poisoning is most often lethal. The ingestion or inhalation of selenium dioxide or selenious acid (found in gun bluing solutions) can cause a dramatic drop in blood pressure, due to its toxic effects on the heart muscle, and a dilation (opening up) of the blood vessels throughout the body, which can lead to cardiac arrest and death. It can cause severe burns to the skin and the lining of the mouth as well as the lungs, where bleeding and pulmonary edema (lungs filling with water) may result. A reddish pigmentation of the teeth, hair, and nails coupled with a garlic-like odor on the breath are typical of acute poisoning.

Chronic poisoning occurs with long-term, low-level exposure. The victim's skin may develop a reddish hue, and a pruritic (itchy) scalp rash may appear. The hair becomes brittle and breaks easily or falls out. The nails become brittle and display red or yellowish white transverse or longitudinal lines. The breath smells of garlic, and the victim may complain of a metallic taste in the mouth. Nausea, vomiting, fatigue, irritability, emotional lability, depression, tremors, and muscle tenderness may also occur.

The diagnosis of selenium poisoning, either in the living or at autopsy, is made by testing the victim's blood and urine for increased selenium levels. At autopsy, findings would likely include congestion in the lungs and kidneys, patchy scarring and enlargement of the heart, edema and swelling of the brain, and a orange-brown discoloration of the skin and internal organs.

For those who survive, treatment consists of stopping any chronic exposure and using intramuscular doses of dimercaprol (also called BAL, or British Anti-Lewisite). BAL acts as a chelating agent by binding the selenium and removing it from the body via the kidneys. The usual schedule is the injection of 3 to 5 milligrams per kilogram of body weight every four hours for two days, every six hours on the third day, and then every twelve hours thereafter for ten days.

For your purposes, either an acute or a chronic poisoning could work, depending on whether you want the character to die right away or slowly over a month or so. Gun bluing solutions contain lethal amounts of selenious acid, and a couple of tablespoons added to food or drink could kill the person in a couple of hours. Adding a little here and there day by day would accomplish a chronic poisoning. The victim would gradually become sicker. His appetite would disappear, his weight would drop, and nausea and vomiting would occur. His hair would fall out, and he would become weak, short of breath, and irritable. His hands would develop a tremor, and he might develop heart failure and pulmonary edema. His doctor might diagnose heart disease or gastroenteritis or even the flu. Selenium poisoning would never enter his mind. He would treat him with digitalis and diuretics or suggest fluids, aspirin, and rest. As the condition progressed, the victim might be hospitalized and then die of progressive heart failure. Since death from heart failure is a common occurrence, the death would likely be written off to plain old heart failure—that is, until your protagonist became suspicious and tracked down the true cause of the victim's demise.

How Quickly Would Someone Die After Drinking Alcohol Laced with Xanax?

Q: One of my characters crushes Xanax tabs and then adds the powder to another's Scotch. Both men have been drinking. Would the Xanax interact quickly with the alcohol to depress the central nervous system? How much should be used to achieve the desired effect? Would there be any immediate reaction to the mix (that is, vomiting)? What would the specific symptoms be as the character slips into unconsciousness, and how soon would death occur?

A: Xanax (alprazolam) is a short-acting sedative in the benzodiazepine family (along with Valium, Halcion, Restoril, Ativan, and others). It is a relatively safe sedative, but when mixed with alcohol, it can be deadly. Of course, it depends on the dosage of both the Xanax and the alcohol as well as the underlying health, size, and age of the victim. People with chronic lung or heart disease are more susceptible, as are the young and the old.

Xanax comes in white oval tablets of .25 milligram (mg), 0.5 mg (peach), and 1 mg (light blue). It also comes in a white oblong 2 mg tablet. It dissolves easily and is well absorbed by the GI tract. It reaches its peak effect about one to two hours after ingestion, but its effects would begin to appear in less than half an hour.

Now to your specific questions:

Yes, it would begin to act quickly—a half hour or perhaps less if the victim consumed a large amount of alcohol beforehand. The victim would become lethargic and have slurred speech, poor coordination, and confusion. He might stagger and even fall. He would speak slowly with a thick tongue, and his words may not make sense. In short, he would appear very intoxicated. He would soon lose consciousness, after which his respirations would decline and finally cease. Death would then follow in a few minutes.

The rapidity with which this process unfolds would depend on many factors, but if you give him an hour, you'll be okay. More is better, but as little as thirty minutes would also work.

One problem with Xanax is that it requires several tablets to do the trick. This depends, of course, on how much alcohol the victim downed. If he is intoxicated before the loaded drink is given, less Xanax is required. If your killer crushes ten of the 2 mg tablets, that should do it. If the victim is already intoxicated, he likely won't notice any alteration in the taste of his drink. This is particularly true if you use some flavored concoction rather than Scotch.

What Substance Can Be Added to a Fire-Eater's "Fuel" to Cause a Sudden and Dramatic Death?

Q: I want to kill off a street performer, a fire-eater in Madrid, by substituting or adding a substance to the clear liquid these people swish in their mouth and then blow out to be ignited. Since they don't actually swallow the liquid, I need something that is very deadly, won't alter the clear nature of the liquid, and hopefully won't be immediately detected when the liquid enters the mouth. Also, I'd like the death to be relatively quick and dramatic.

A: Cyanide is quick, nasty, and very effective. It kills instantly. The person will suddenly become short of breath, may clutch his chest as if having a heart attack, may suffer a seizure, may foam at the mouth, and will definitely fall over dead. Since cyanide is a metabolic poison, which means it poisons the body's cells so that they cannot use oxygen, even if some bystander began CPR or other life-saving measure, the victim would die anyway. Effective CPR would supply blood and oxygen to the tissues, but the cyanide would prevent the tissues from using the oxygen, so death would be the result regardless.

Cyanide comes as a powder in the form of potassium cyanide (KCN) and sodium cyanide (NaCN). It dissolves easily in most liquids and requires only a tiny amount to be deadly. It has a slight bitter almond smell and taste, which would be undetectable in the flammable liquid.

In your scenario the fire-eater would take a mouthful of the liquid and within a few seconds clutch his throat or chest, spit out the liquid, gasp for breath, cry out for help, collapse to the ground (with or without a seizure), and die quickly.

One caveat: The person handling the cyanide should not let it contact his skin since it is readily absorbed through the skin. The use of rubber gloves would be safest.

Cyanide is used in metal plating and tanning and can be obtained from many chemical supply houses or stolen by your villain from any place that plates jewelry or uses it in other ways.

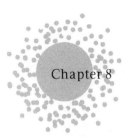

Chapter 8

MEDICAL MURDER

How Can Someone Who Is Undergoing Heart Surgery Be Murdered?

Q: I need help with a hospital scene. The bad guys decide to execute a very successful and powerful enemy while he is in the hospital undergoing a heart bypass operation. The plan is a strike against the hospital's primary and redundant power sources, effectively imperiling all patients in the hospital or wing, not just the intended. Now the questions: How does one take down the hospital power grid and its backup systems? Where is the most ticklish point of the bypass surgery to have a power loss?

A: Most hospitals have backup generators that switch on automatically when the power supply is interrupted. I suspect that most of these systems are computer controlled, so your villain can approach the problem in several ways.

He could attack the computers and effectively shut down both the main power and the backup generator at will. A good hacker could tamper with the control program, and then they could be shut off on command—maybe by remote control with a wireless modem.

Or he could disengage or disable the backup and then cut the main power supply by severing the hospital's incoming power line or knocking out the local power station. That would deal with the power supply to the entire hospital but would not completely resolve your problem.

In cardiac surgery the patient is typically placed on a heart-lung machine, which acts as his heart and lungs by circulating and oxygenating the blood while the operation is being performed. The pump is dependent on a power supply to function, but these gadgets have both an internal backup battery supply as well as a hand-crank system for just such power loss situations. This means that your bad guys would have to tamper with the heart-lung pump itself. They would need to damage or disconnect the battery or its cables, or mangle the gears and pulleys that are part of the hand-crank system.

These heart-lung machines are typically kept within the surgical suites (operating rooms) of the hospital, an area that has restricted access. Still, someone with knowledge of the layout could sneak in, especially at night when fewer staff members are on duty.

Or an insider could be involved. The best person for this would be either someone in the bioengineering department (called biotechs for short) or one of the technicians who run the heart-lung machine (called pump techs).

The biotechs maintain and repair most of the medical gadgetry in the hospital. Some techs can fix anything, while others have to call in repairmen from the various manufacturers or independent biomedical repair companies more frequently. Your tech could be the insider, or the accomplice could be the outside tech he called in. Either would work.

Most major medical centers have pump techs on staff, while smaller hospitals contract to outside companies for techs who come in and work on a case-by-case basis. The in-house techs have easy access to the machines any time they aren't in use. For the contracted tech, things would be more difficult. Since he goes into the OR only when a case is scheduled and since there are always several nurses and operating room technicians around preparing for surgery, he would have to be fairly slick to tamper with the backup systems. It's possible, just more difficult.

The best time to attack the power supply would be during the operation. That is when the patient/victim would be most vulnerable. If your villains could accomplish their tampering after the patient/victim is "on bypass," on the heart-lung machine, a loss of power would be potentially fatal. During the surgery, the heart is stopped by a combination of cooling the blood and delivering a large dose of potassium. (We call this "cold cardioplegia.") After the operation, the heart-lung machine rewarms the blood and washes out the potassium; then the heart resumes beating on its own. This takes ten to fifteen minutes or more to accomplish.

If the power and the backup systems failed, the surgeon would be left with only internal cardiac massage to maintain blood flow and keep the patient alive. Internal cardiac massage is simply squeezing the heart rhythmically with your hand. The surgeon would then begin giving the patient warmed blood and intravenous fluids in an attempt to rewarm the patient and wash out the potassium. This would be difficult and could take as much as half an hour to an hour without the aid of a functioning heart-lung machine. But this is what they get the big bucks for. Failure to do so would certainly result in the patient's death, which is what you want.

Of course, the patient/victim could survive this event or not, as you wish. Either way is plausible. If he is to survive, the surgeon must give the warmed blood and fluids rapidly, close up any of the coronary arteries he had been working on, close up the patient's chest, and get him to the ICU as quickly as possible. Meanwhile, the biomedical people would work frantically to repair the machine.

This is good stuff, an exciting scene.

What Dose of Morphine Would Kill a Man Undergoing Cancer Treatment?

Q: My victim is in the final stages of metastatic lung cancer and is taking morphine intravenously at home, administered by a pump. For a 145-pound male who is seventy-six years of age, what might a typical dosage be? Would twice that amount cause a deadly overdose?

A: Metastatic lung cancer can be a very painful disease. Cancers that originate in the lung often metastasize (spread) to the liver, the brain, and the bones. In medical jargon these metastatic lesions are often referred to as "mets." Brain mets tend to enlarge within the closed space inside the skull and also cause swelling of the surrounding brain tissue. The net effect is a rise in intracranial (inside the skull or cranium) pressure. This can cause severe continuous headaches. Mets to bones such as the ribs and the spine can be extremely painful. For this reason narcotics such as morphine sulfate (MS), Demerol, Dilaudid, and others are commonly used. In an individual with terminal cancer the risk of addiction is of little concern.

The chosen analgesic (pain reliever) may be given by intermittent injections or by use of one of the automated methods. Continuous infusion pumps and patient-controlled analgesia (PCA) are commonly employed in this circumstance. The former is by definition a continuous infusion of fluid containing the sedating drug, usually MS. PCA is a system of IV delivery that allows the patient to control the timing of delivery within preprescribed parameters. Here, a syringe filled with the MS is placed in an automatic injector that is attached to the patient's IV line. The injector delivers a prescribed amount of the drug when the patient depresses a hand-held button. Parameters are set to limit the amount that can be requested per hour. Within these limits, the patient may use as much or as little as he feels is necessary.

As with many medications, the dosing of MS is determined by the patient's weight. The dosing schedule in most patients ranges from 0.2 to 0.4 milligram (mg) per kilogram (kg) of body weight per hour and then is titrated (a gradual increase in dose) upward as needed. Since one kilogram equals 2.2 pounds, your 145-pound (66 kg) patient would require approximately 13 to 26 mg per hour. However, in patients who have been on the continuous drip or PCA for weeks or months, tolerance to the drug develops, just as it does in addicts. Therefore, larger and larger doses are needed to obtain the same sedating and pain-relieving effect. Some patients in this situation require doses as high as 500 mg per hour, which is enough to kill even the strongest person not habituated to the drug.

In large doses MS depresses respiration and drops the blood pressure. If enough is given, the recipient will stop breathing, his blood pressure will fall to dangerously low levels, and he will die from apnea (absence of breathing) and shock. The dose required to kill someone depends on the rate of delivery, the underlying medical condition of the victim, and whether the victim has developed tolerance to the drug.

Doubling the dose at any given level may or may not be enough to be lethal. For example, if a patient was receiving 60 mg per hour and the rate was doubled to 120 mg per hour, it probably wouldn't do him in, though it certainly could do in a debilitated man with terminal lung cancer. Raising it to 240 mg per hour (quadruple) probably would work. A half hour to two or three hours at this increased rate may be required to do the victim in.

On the other hand, if given as a single injection, an extra 20 to 40 mg might be enough. Since the person on a drip of 60 mg per hour receives 1 mg per minute, giving 20 to 40 mg over a few seconds is a large increase in dose and would probably work. MS works rapidly, within a minute or so, when given as a bolus (a single, rapid injection), so you are actually increasing the dose from 1 mg per minute to 41 mg per minute—a huge increase that would likely cause apnea and shock almost instantaneously.

So either markedly increasing the rate of administration (by increasing the drip rate or the concentration of the drug per cubic centimeter of fluid, or both) or giving a bolus of the drug would accomplish your goal in this situation.

Additionally, patients with lung cancer often have sicker lungs, not just from the cancer itself but from surgery that removes part or all of one lung and radiation therapy or chemotherapy, which may damage the good lung tissue. In this case, even smaller amounts might work.

I suggest either quadrupling the rate or giving 40 mg as an IV bolus, depending on which scenario fits your story best.

Can a Transfusion Reaction Be Used for Murder?

Q: In my story an elderly and seriously ill man is murdered by a nurse who switches the blood he is to receive, causing a reaction that kills him. How does this reaction occur, and what symptoms would the victim have?

A: Transfusion reactions come in many varieties. They may be as mild as a rash or perhaps chills and fevers, or be so severe as to cause death. First let's look at why these reactions occur.

The red blood cells (RBCs) are the carriers of oxygen from the lungs to the tissues and of carbon dioxide from the tissues to the lungs. This is accomplished by using the hemoglobin inside the RBCs. The RBCs also have antigens on their surface, and they are at the root of transfusion reactions.

These antigens are designated either A or B. From these our blood-typing system (ABO system) has been derived. Type A blood has only A antigens, type B only B antigens, type AB both, and type O neither.

Simple, so far. But the serum of the blood (the liquid part) also carries antibodies. It is the reaction of these antibodies with the antigens of the transfused blood that causes problems.

Type A serum (that is, the serum of people with type A blood) has anti-B antibodies. Type B has anti-A antibodies. Type AB has neither. Type O has both anti-A and anti-B antibodies.

Type	Antigens on RBCs	Antibodies in Serum
A	A	Anti-B
B	B	Anti-A
AB	AB	None
O	Neither	Anti-A and Anti-B

Reactions occur when blood with the right antigen is given to a person with the its corresponding antibody. For example, if a type A person (who has anti-B antibodies in the serum) receives type B blood (which has the B antigen on its RBCs) or type AB blood (which has both A and B antigens), an adverse reaction will occur because the anti-B antibodies in the recipient's serum will react with the B antigens on the transfused RBCs. This is a transfusion reaction. The result is agglutination, or clumping, of the blood cells and the release of several harmful chemicals that cause the symptoms and signs of this basically "allergic" reaction.

It gets more complicated than this because there are other antigen/antibody problems with blood matching such as the well-known Rh factor, which is either positive or negative, and many others, mostly named after the physicians that discovered them. Your blood type is typically expressed only in terms of the ABO and Rh systems. For example, a person who is A-positive has type A blood and the Rh factor antigen is present, while a person who is O-negative has type O blood and the Rh factor is absent.

Because of the multitude of potentially problematic antigens, blood is typed and cross-matched prior to transfusion. This tests the blood that is to be given directly against the recipient's blood to determine if any antigens and antibodies exist that might cause the blood to be incompatible and thus lead to reactions. In very emergent situations such as gunshots, stabbings, or automobile accidents where the victim is bleeding to death and there isn't time to do a complete cross-match, type-specific blood is given. A person's blood type can be determined in a few minutes, but cross-matching may take hours. In these cases a type A person receives type A blood, and everyone hopes for the best.

In your story I would suggest that you have your victim be type A and have the nurse switch the blood to type B. This would definitely cause a reaction. The patient would develop fever, chills, and a diffuse, irregular red rash over his entire body. This could begin within minutes or be delayed for a few hours. This type of reaction would not likely result in death.

However, your victim could develop a full-blown anaphylactic allergic reaction, which would be the above symptoms plus swelling of the face, lips, hands, and feet, shortness of breath, low blood pressure, and severe shock with pallor, cold and clammy skin, and a bluish tinge (called cyanosis) to his lips, fingers, and toes. He would ultimately suffer cardiac arrest and death. Since this represents the severest form of allergic reaction, anaphylaxis would develop fairly quickly after the blood was infused.

If the victim survived an anaphylactic reaction, there is a strong probability that his kidneys would be severely and irreparably damaged, requiring dialysis. This damage results from the kidneys' attempt to filter the clumped RBCs from the blood. The iron found in the hemoglobin molecules of the RBCs is particularly toxic to the kidney tissues.

Can a Bee Sting Kit Be Altered to Result in the Death of the User?

Q: I have a scene in which someone who is allergic to bee stings dies after being given a shot from his bee sting kit. Is there a substance that when combined with medicine in the bee sting remedy would prove fatal?

A: The deadly allergic reaction that follows bee stings in susceptible individuals is called anaphylaxis. It is a severe allergic reaction that causes spasm of the lung's bronchial tubes (breathing airways), which basically causes a severe asthmatic attack with shortness of breath and wheezing. Anaphylaxis also is associated with a profound drop in blood pressure, leading to shock. Without treatment, death can quickly follow.

Common causative agents of anaphylaxis and other allergic reactions include antibiotics (penicillin, sulfa), local anesthetics (lidocaine, procaine), antisera (gamma globulin, tetanus), foods (nuts, shellfish, eggs), iodine (used in certain X-ray exams), and insect stings (yellow jacket wasps, honeybees, fire ants). When an allergic individual is exposed to the allergenic substance, the reaction may be immediate and profound.

The emergent treatment is an injection of epinephrine (adrenaline), which is the substance in the bee sting kits that allergic persons should keep on hand. Epinephrine reverses many of the allergic processes immediately. The person is then transported to the hospital, where further treatment is carried out that typically consists of oxygen, medications for blood pressure support, antihistamines (such as Benadryl), and steroids.

One way to do the victim in would be to replace the epinephrine with water. He would then succumb to the bee sting.

Another way would be to tamper with the concentration of the epinephrine. Reducing it would probably not work since the net effect would be a partial treatment, which might be enough to allow the victim to reach the hospital. It would be better to increase the concentration.

Epinephrine is basically speed. If given in large amounts, it can cause marked elevation of the blood pressure and deadly changes in cardiac rhythm that can kill almost instantly. The emergency bee sting kits are called Epipen Auto-Injectors and contain 0.3 cc of epinephrine at a 1:1000 dilution. This means that each cc of the medication contains 1 milligram (mg) of epinephrine. Thus, the delivery of 0.3 cc yields a dose of 0.3 mg.

Increasing the dose by a factor of five or ten—a dose of 1.5 to 3 mg—could cause the desired result (cardiac arrhythmia and death), especially if given intravenously. In your scenario, giving either multiple injections (not practical) or tampering with the drug concentration in one of the injectors would do this. Substituting a more concentrated solution of epinephrine could work. The beauty of this approach is that no new drug is required, and the coroner might assume that the victim died from the standard dose of epinephrine, which can rarely happen, or from the allergic reaction itself. Of course, if the coroner tested the residue in the auto-injector, he would likely be able to determine that the concentration of the drug had been altered. But maybe not.

If you want to add another drug, any speedlike product would do the trick, since the effect of the epinephrine and the other drug would be additive. Many of these are readily available. Cocaine (basically a speedball when mixed with an amphetamine such as epinephrine), crystal methamphetamine, and perhaps the rave drug Ecstasy, which is methylenedioxymethamphetamine, would work.

The effect of this would be to raise the blood pressure and heart rate severely and rapidly, which could precipitate a heart attack. Also, these drugs can cause spasm of the coronary arteries, which could lead to a heart attack. Or the combination could cause a fatal change in heart rhythm. Cocaine and crystal meth are notorious for causing spasm of the coronary arteries and for precipitating deadly arrhythmias. In this case immediately after injection of the speedball the victim would feel warm and flushed, his heart would pound, and he might experience chest tightness or pressure, clutch his chest, and collapse. Or in the case of a sudden arrhythmia he might simply collapse with no warning symptoms at all.

Can Insulin Be Used for Murder? How?

Q: For my story, I need to know how easy it would be to kill someone with insulin. I know it can't be taken by mouth, but can it be given in an IV? Would the insulin overdose be detected in an autopsy? How much insulin would it take to kill an adult who is not diabetic?

A: Insulin, which is produced in the pancreas by specialized cells called islet cells, is necessary for life. These islet cells constantly "read" the sugar level in the blood and secrete insulin as needed. The cells of the body require insulin in order to take in sugar from the bloodstream, metabolize it (break it down), and produce energy.

Diabetics often have a deficiency of insulin or a faulty system for release of insulin from the pancreas. Untreated, this leads to elevated blood sugars, altered cellular sugar utilization, and a host of problems including diabetic coma and death.

Excess insulin causes the rapid uptake of sugars by some cells and leaves none for the brain, thus leading to a hypoglycemic (low blood sugar) coma, brain damage, or death. Rare insulin-producing tumors can also cause profound hypoglycemia. And diabetics who give themselves too much insulin or don't eat enough after taking insulin can end up in the same situation.

Since the brain, heart, and other organs need sugar for the energy to function, when the blood sugar level drops below 60 or so, symptoms of hunger, nausea, sleepiness, headache, and confusion appear. When the sugar falls further (30 to 50, say) all these symptoms worsen, followed by coma, brain damage, and ultimately death. Also, cardiac arrhythmias may appear and lead to death.

Now to your questions.

No, insulin cannot be taken orally. Digestive enzymes that break down food also digest insulin. Yes, insulin can be given by IV or added to an IV infusion of fluids. We do this from time to time to control very brittle (hard to control) diabetics who are in extreme circumstances.

For your purposes an IV "push" dose of 50 to 100 units of insulin would do just about anyone in. A lesser amount probably would, too, but to be sure, 100 is a good number. It would work in less than a minute or two. It could also be given intramuscularly (injected into a muscle) or subcutaneously (injected beneath the skin, which is the method diabetics use to give themselves daily doses) and would have a slightly slower (fifteen to twenty minutes or less before the person lost consciousness) but still deadly effect.

Yes, the coroner would be able to detect the excess insulin and the very low blood sugar at the postmortem exam. Of course, if the victim was a diabetic, he may write it off to an unfortunate incident. This happens to insulin-dependent diabetics all too often. Since your victim is not a diabetic, the presence of high insulin levels and low blood sugar would prompt a search for an insulin-secreting tumor of the pancreas, and when none was found, homicide would become the likely cause.

Would Denying a Diabetic Insulin Cause Death or Just Illness?

Q: For my story, I want to know whether a murder could be committed by substituting water for the insulin of a diabetic. What would happen to the victim, and how

long would it take? Would the coroner be able to determine what had happened?

A: Yes, a murder could be carried out in this fashion, but the victim would have to be an insulin-dependent diabetic. Let me
explain.

Diabetes is separated into two broad types. One is called adult-
onset, non-insulin-dependent, or Type 2 diabetes. The pancreas in
this situation produces insulin, though usually in reduced amounts.
These people do not require insulin and are typically managed
with diet and possibly medications. The drugs used in this circumstance either enhance the body's sensitivity to insulin or promote
insulin production and release by the pancreas.

The second type of diabetes is called juvenile-onset, insulin-
dependent, or Type 1 diabetes. The pancreas in these people produces little if any insulin, and they require insulin to survive. Often
when you hear on the news that a child is missing and needs to be
found quickly because he or she needs important medicines, the
problem is juvenile diabetes.

In a Type 1 diabetic, tampering with or diluting the insulin or
preventing the victim from getting it could lead to diabetic
ketoacidosis, coma, and death. It may take a few hours or several
days for the victim to get into trouble, depending on how much
insulin is needed, how severe the diabetes is, and other factors.

The symptoms of rising blood sugar and impending diabetic
coma are fatigue, shortness of breath, nausea, thirst, excess urination
(the high sugar in the blood is filtered through the kidneys and acts
as a diuretic, causing a sudden increase in urine volume and leading
to dehydration), lethargy, somnolence, confusion, and finally coma
and death.

At autopsy the M.E. would find elevated blood sugar and acido-
sis, which would lead him to conclude that the victim died from
diabetic ketoacidosis. He would not be able to determine why the
victim didn't take his insulin or why he took an inadequate

amount. That said, the M.E. would not only examine the victim but also all the evidence collected at the scene that might bear on the cause and manner of death. He could test the insulin bottle found in the victim's house and discover that it had been diluted, which might lead him to consider homicide as the cause of death.

Is There a Lethal Substance That When Given to a Patient Might Appear to Be a Hospital Blunder Rather than a Homicide?

Q: I have a killer (fictional, of course) who is attempting to murder a hospitalized patient by putting some material through the IV while he sleeps. What readily available substance could he use to make the hit look like a hospital blunder rather than a homicide?

A: In the hospital setting, many drugs are available that would surely fit your story requirements.

Any of the muscular paralytic agents would work. This class of drugs paralyzes all the muscles, including those used for respiration. The victim would stop breathing and die. Since these drugs work on all the muscles, he would not be able to move or speak or cry for help. Anectine and Pavulon are examples. Anectine (succinylcholine chloride) comes in multidose vials of 10 cc that contain 20 milligrams (mg) per cc of the drug. Give the entire 200 mg through the IV and paralysis will occur in a matter of seconds. Pavulon (pancuronium bromide) comes in 10 cc vials with 1 mg per cc of the drug. Again, give the entire vial intravenously.

Almost any narcotic or barbiturate (barbie) would also work. In large doses they depress and can even stop respiration, and they are available in most hospital wards and/or pharmacies.

Common narcotics include Morphine (MS, or morphine sulfate), Demerol (meperidine hydrochloride), and Dilaudid (hydromorphone hydrochloride). Once again, overkill is the operative word, so very large doses should be given intravenously to assure the desired effect. For MS give 100 mg; Demerol, 250 mg; and Dilaudid, 20 mg.

The two most common injectable barbies are pentobarbital (trade name Nembutal) and sodium phenobarbital. Giving 2 to 5 grams of pentobarbital or 500 to 1000 milligrams (½ to 1 gram) of phenobarbital would do anyone in.

The problem with all of these drugs is that they are traceable. And since they work by stopping respiration, it would take a couple of minutes for the victim to die, which allows time for the nurse to discover the person is in trouble and begin lifesaving measures. Thus, the patient would have to be on the ward and not in the ICU or Coronary Care Unit where they have cardiac and respiratory monitors that sound a warning if respiration drops. On the wards these devices are used less often, and the nurses aren't always in eye contact with the patients, so the victim could die before anyone knew about it.

Another option would be injecting potassium chloride (KCl) intravenously. This is the truly lethal part of lethal injection executions. It stops the heart immediately. A dose of 50 to 100 milli-equilivents (meq) pushed rapidly intravenously will kill anyone. Milliequivalents is a chemistry term that would be very difficult to explain, and you don't really need to know this to craft a credible scene. It comes in vials that contain 40 meq per cc. It is easily available in a hospital, and right or wrong is often left lying around. It is commonly given to patients with low potassium levels as part of their IV fluid infusion—at slower rates than an IV push, of course. This would be traceable in that a high potassium level in the blood would be found at autopsy. That said, it could still be written off as a medical error, and the nurse could get blamed.

A better bet would be to use a drug that the victim is already taking and simply give him a large dose. This could easily be deemed a medical error. For example, if the victim had heart disease and was taking one of the antiarrhythmic drugs (commonly used medications that treat abnormal cardiac rhythms), giving a large dose could kill him, and finding a high level in the victim's blood at autopsy might be interpreted as physician or nurse error. Examples of these drugs would be quinidine and procainamide. Give 1,000 mg of either by rapid IV injection, and the victim's heart would come to a standstill in a minute or two.

Another possibility would be digitalis, a common cardiac medication. Digitalis is manufactured under several trade names. The most common is Digoxin, and the typical daily oral dose is 0.25 mg. Giving 2 mg intravenously would kill almost anyone in a few minutes by causing a deadly change in cardiac rhythm. Again, this could appear to be a nursing error.

What Drugs or Medicines Will Become Deadly When Combined with an MAO Inhibitor?

Q: I have a female character who recently had a face-lift. She does fine through the surgery and is released with antiinflammatory and pain medications. Two days later she dies because of a severe reaction to her medications. An autopsy discovers that someone substituted one of her medications for something dangerous. I was thinking of MAOI. Will this work? Can you give me the names of the medications prescribed and the substitute that would kill her?

A: The answer is very complex, but I'll try to keep it as simple as possible.

The monoamine oxidase inhibitors (MAOIs) are a strange group of drugs and very treacherous. So much so that most physicians avoid using them, and many of the older MAOIs are off the market. However, some still exist and are used in the treatment of depression.

Nardil (phenelzine sulfate) is still around and is a very potent MAO inhibitor. It comes as a shiny orange pill with "P-D 270" stamped on it in brown lettering. The tablet contains 15 mg of the active compound.

The physiology of MAO inhibitor action is very complex, and I won't bore you with the details. The important thing is that if these drugs are given with certain other drugs and foods, severe and potentially lethal reactions can occur.

The most dangerous drugs to combine with the MAOIs are the sympathomimetics. These are the adrenaline or speedlike drugs. Cocaine, epinephrine (often used with local anesthetics to lessen bleeding; an example is lidocaine with epinephrine that dentists use frequently), pseudoephedrine (found in Sudafed and Actifed), amphetamines (found in nearly every diet pill), and certain serotonergic drugs can cause serious reactions. Most decongestants, asthma inhalers, cold medicines, and diet pills contain these or similar compounds that can lead to deadly interactions.

Also, foods that contain high concentrations of tyramine, L-tryptophan, or dopamine can cause dangerous reactions. These include aged cheeses, dry sausages (pepperoni, hard salami), pickled herring, fava beans, beer, wine, liver, yeast extract, and even caffeine and chocolate.

Now you can see why the MAOIs have fallen into disfavor. There are simply too many substances that can interact with them and cause lethal complications.

The most deadly reactions include the following:

Hypertensive crisis: The blood pressure (BP) shoots up rapidly to very high levels—250 to 300 over 100 to 130 wouldn't be unusual. This can cause confusion, disorientation, headache, blurred vision, seizures, loss of consciousness. It may lead to a stroke, a bleed into the brain, or a heart attack. Treatment is the administration of 5 mg of phentolamine intravenously to lower the BP rapidly.

Hyperpyrexia: The acute and severe elevation of body temperature. Temperatures of 106 to 108 and higher may occur. Any time the body temperature rises above 106, brain cells begin dying in fairly short order and death follows. Treatment is an ice water bath.

In your scenario it would be easy to substitute two of the victim's medications with Nardil and any of the currently available diet pills such as Meridia (silbutramine hydrochloride monohydrate, which is supplied in capsules: blue/yellow is 5 mg; blue/white is 10 mg; yellow/white is 15 mg) or Fastin (phentermine hydrochloride, which is supplied in 15 and 30 mg capsules). For the most potent lethal effect, begin the Nardil several days (two to eight or more) before giving the diet pill. A hypertensive crisis could ensue rapidly, and the victim would suffer a stroke or cardiac arrest. This could occur within twenty to thirty minutes or up to several hours after the medication was taken.

The victim would develop a severe headache, blurred vision, dizziness, nausea, shortness of breath, confusion and disorientation, perhaps chest pain, perhaps a nosebleed from the high BP, and then collapse and die. These events could occur over several minutes to a few hours, whichever works for you.

As I said, this is a complex topic but an interesting question.

Follow-up Question and Answer

How Does a Physician Distinguish Between a Drug-Induced Fever and One from an Infectious Process?

Q: Could the elevated temperature be misdiagnosed as an infection at first? What would an autopsy pick up in such a situation?

A: Yes, the elevated temperature could lead the M.D. down the wrong road and probably would. An adage in medicine is that "common things occur commonly." A person with very high fever and lethargy or coma or seizures or other neurologic symptoms would be assumed to have an infection first—particularly an infection of the brain such as meningitis or a brain abscess. Only after these were ruled out would other things be considered. And in the real world a drug interaction with MAOIs in a patient who wasn't taking those medications would not likely even come to mind. Therefore, it would be found only if the M.D. taking care of the victim obtained a drug screen and it appeared there.

The tests to rule out the infections mentioned above could include blood cultures, CT or MRI brain scans, a spinal tap to examine the cerebrospinal fluid for infectious critters and white blood cells, and an EEG (brain wave test), for starters.

In your scenario the victim could collapse or suffer a seizure and be taken to the ER, where her temperature would be found to be 106 and the workup for a brain infection would then ensue. Her blood pressure would likely be very elevated, which can also happen in brain infections if the brain swells and the intracranial pressure (pressure inside the skull) rises. The victim could die in a few hours, which would automatically make it a coroner's case. Anyone who dies within twenty-four hours of hospital admission must at some level be reviewed by the coroner.

The M.D. wouldn't know if the cause of death was indeed an infection or not. The coroner would perform a postmortem exam, find no signs of infection, and would then await the toxicology and other tests before determining the true cause of death. This may take a few days.

Can a Patient Be Killed by the Rapid Injection of Potassium Intravenously?

Q: Does this sound like a credible way for my villain to kill a hospitalized patient? An insulin syringe filled with potassium chloride (40 meq per cc) is injected quickly into an IV line just above the point where the IV's

needle enters the skin. Would there be too much dilution from the IV solution already in the line? If it
worked, could this look like a hospital accident if the
victim was receiving treatment for dehydration, exposure, and malnourishment? Would he be getting something like potassium chloride to elevate his electrolytes
anyway?

A: Absolutely. Patients suffering from dehydration and malnutri-
tion often receive IV fluids, which are typically D5½ normal saline
with 40 milliequivalents of KCL per liter. This means a liter (1000
cc) bag of saline which has half the salt (NaCl) of "normal" blood
(thus "½ Normal Saline") to which 40 meq of potassium chloride
(KCl) has been added. It is typically given at 100 to 200 cc per
hour, which means the potassium is going at a rate of 4 to 8 meq
per hour (40 meq in 1000 cc yields 4 meq per 100 cc).

Giving KCl faster than 20 meq per hour is dangerous, so the
above flow rate is well below that. Pushing 100 meq of KCl intravenously is obviously way above this, and dilution is nonexistent in
"IV push" administration. This dose would stop anyone's heart in
seconds.

One caveat: Concentrated KCl like this burns severely when
given, so the patient/victim would react unless he was in a coma or
very heavily sedated. Of course he will die quickly, but he would
yell out before he fades to black because it burns that severely. Factor this into your plot, and you'll be okay.

Options: The victim could be in a coma or sedated or restrained,
and the killer could hold a pillow over his face while giving the
KCL. Nurses could be distracted by a Code Blue or an unruly
patient at the other end of the hall. The fire alarm could be trig-
gered to create confusion.

If Someone with Tuberculosis Is Smothered, Would There Be Blood on the Pillow?

Q: How would someone look who had been suffocated with a pillow? If the person also had tuberculosis, would the pillow have signs of blood that had been coughed up?

A: Asphyxia by pillow suffocation leaves less evidence than manual or ligature strangulation because bruises or abrasions on the neck are not present. However, asphyxiations of all types typically result in petechial hemorrhages (also called petechiae) in the conjunctivae of the eyes (the pink mucous membranes that line the eyelids and surround the eyeball). The petechiae are small bright red dots or splotches, usually pinpoint or slightly larger in size. When these are found, some form of asphyxiation is likely, and your M.E. or sleuth would determine this quickly.

In addition, most victims of asphyxia have a deep purple color to their skin, particularly the head, neck, and upper body. Also, if the victim struggles, he may bite his tongue, sometimes severely, or may have the attacker's skin and blood under his fingernails.

As far as TB goes, bleeding would be unlikely but possible. TB is an infection of the lungs caused by *mycobacterium tuberculosis.* This bacterium causes the formation of tubercles (also called granulomas) in the lungs. These are basically small nodules (small round lumps or clumps), microscopic to pinpoint in size, scattered throughout the lungs. They are composed of the bacteria and the various types of white blood cells sent to fight the infection. These tubercles are the body's attempt to wall off or contain the infection.

Occasionally these tubercles will caseate (break down or liquefy), and if so, they may bleed. The patient will then cough up sputum streaked with blood. We call this hemoptysis. Rarely does the person have severe bleeding.

In your scenario the struggle for air could result in bleeding, but it would likely be streaks of blood, not overt or massive bleeding. The pillow could have streaky bloodstains on it.

Part III

Tracking the Perp

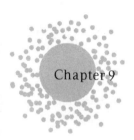

Chapter 9

THE POLICE AND THE CRIME SCENE

What Does the Wound from a Close-Range Gunshot Look Like?

Q: If a young man is shot at close range in the temple and is found within a two-hour time period, what would the wound look like? Simply a hole? Would it have bruising around it?

A: When a gun is fired, the muzzle expels more than the bullet. Burned and unburned powder residue and the hot gases produced by the detonated powder are also released (Figure 17). Each of these can alter the resulting wound pattern and may allow the medical examiner to determine the distance between the muzzle and the victim.

The anatomy of the entrance wound depends on how close the muzzle is to the skin. If it is several feet away, the entrance wound would be a small hole, smaller than the bullet due to the elastic quality of skin (Figure 18a). There would be a blue-black bruising effect in a halo around the entry point (called an "abrasion collar") and some black smudging where the skin literally wipes the bullet clean of the burned powder, grime, and oil residue it picks up during its travel down the barrel. This smudging is often easily wiped away with a wet cloth.

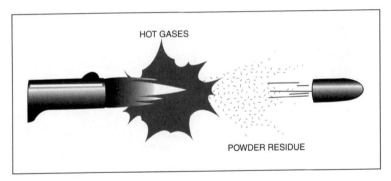

FIGURE 17. MATERIALS EXPELLED FROM A GUN MUZZLE
The explosion of the shell's gunpowder forces the bullet, burned and unburned powder particles, and hot gases from the muzzle. Each of these can leave evidence that helps determine the distance between the muzzle and the victim.

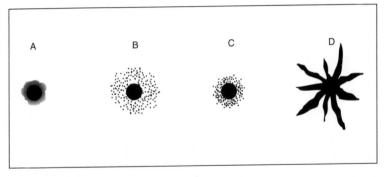

FIGURE 18. THE ANATOMY OF A GUNSHOT WOUND
The entrance wound produced by a gunshot varies depending on how close the muzzle is to the victim. From a distance of several feet the wound will be a small hole with a surrounding abrasion collar (A). If closer, there will also be stippling, or "tattooing," of the skin due to burned and unburned powder residue (B). Closer still, and the stippling will be more compact, and some degree of charring of the skin is likely (C). A contact wound produces a characteristic "stellate" pattern (D).

If the muzzle is closer, there may also be "tattooing" or stippling of the skin (Figure 18b). This is due to burned and unburned powder as well as small pieces of the bullet that are discharged from the muzzle. These tiny particles embed in the skin and/or cause tiny hemorrhages (red dots of blood within the skin) in a speckled or splattered pattern around the wound. These cannot be wiped off because the particles are actually embedded (tattooed) into the skin.

If the muzzle is held very close to the skin, the tattooing pattern is more dense and clustered near the wound since there is less distance for the bullet and powder fragments to fan out (Figure 18c). Also, there will be some charring of the skin due to the hot gases of the muzzle blast.

If the muzzle is held against the skin (contact wound), the actual entrance wound may be larger than the bullet, and the charring is likely to be worse. It will also be more ragged and irregular, and often takes on a "stellate" (starlike) pattern (Figure 18d). This is particularly true if the contact wound is over a bone such as the skull in your scenario. This is due to the explosive gases actually tearing the skin around the muzzle as they follow the path of least resistance. The expanding gases cannot expand the gun barrel or the bone, so they escape laterally by tearing through the layers of the skin.

The exit wound would be large and irregular since the bullet would pass through both sides of the skull, and typically each time a bullet strikes bone, it becomes more flattened, misshapen, or mushroomed. This leads to large, irregular exit wounds.

Follow-up Questions and Answers:

Will a Bullet Fired at Close Range Exit the Skull, and If So, Will the M.E. Be Able to Use It for Ballistic Analysis?

Q1 : Whether the victim is shot at close range or from several feet away, would the bullet exit the skull?

A1 : Your choice. It could or it could not. These things are very unpredictable, and either way is realistic. The physical parameters that determine whether the bullet exits the skull would include the size and weight (caliber) of the bullet, whether the bullet was a hollow point or another type, whether the bullet was jacketed with metal, Teflon, or some other durable coating, the muzzle velocity (the speed the bullet is traveling), the thickness of the cranium (skull bone), the angle at which the bullet struck the skull, and a few other factors. A large, soft, low-speed, hollow-point bullet would be less likely to pass completely through the skull than would a small, high-velocity, Teflon-coated one.

Q2: If the bullet does exit the skull, would there be a way for the pathologist to determine what type of ammo was used?

A2: Unless the bullet was very severely damaged by the skull and the wall or whatever it embedded in, the ballistics people could probably tell the type of ammo and maybe find some rifling grooves for comparison if the weapon or other bullets from the same gun were found. On the other hand, the bullet could be so fractured, flattened, or distorted that little of use could be gleaned. If the bullet wasn't found, an experienced M.E. might be able to guess the caliber and type of ammunition used from the nature of the bullet track through the skull and brain, but a definitive answer would likely be impossible. Again, it is your choice as to whether the bullet is identifiable or not. Either is realistic.

Can Stored Blood Be Used to Stage a Death?

Q: If someone removed and stored his own blood and later used it to stage his death, would the coroner be able to tell that the blood wasn't fresh? The scene I have in mind is a car over a cliff and into the ocean. No body would be found, but the victim's blood would be on the glass and upholstery, leading the police to conclude the body must have washed out to sea. Would the blood need a preservative to keep it from clotting? Could it also be frozen and thawed? Would the fact that the blood was stored or thawed show up in the forensic tests? Would the salt water interfere with DNA matching?

A: The victim could remove his own blood and either use an anticoagulant (any substance that prevents blood from clotting) such as EDTA or let it clot, then refrigerate or freeze it. In a typical crime scene such as in a room or an accident on dry land, the M.E. might be able to determine if the blood had clotted beforehand by looking at the microscopic organization of the clot. Its architecture may make him suspicious that the blood had clotted before it reached the scene. For example, a large clot of blood lying on the carpet with no corona of blood soaking the carpet around it may look as though it was simply dumped there rather than bled there, which of course would be the case.

He might also be able to determine if unclotted blood had been frozen. He would look for fracturing of red blood cells, which occurs during freezing. Also, since blood clots very quickly after it leaves the body, if the M.E. found a pool of blood that hadn't clotted, he would likely conclude that some form of anticoagulant was present and thus the scene had been staged. He would then test the blood for the presence of an anticoagulant.

If the blood was flash frozen and later thawed out and dumped at the scene, where it would then clot, the M.E. would probably not be able to determine if the blood had been frozen. The clotting process itself fragments and destroys most of the red blood cells (RBCs) so that any fragmentation of the RBCs would be assumed to have occurred due to the clotting.

The M.E. might not be able to make a clear determination in any case, however.

In the scenario you describe, the car would be in the water, and probably beneath it, and this fact would change the evidence dramatically. Most of the blood would wash away so that the M.E.

would be dealing with residual stains on the seats, doors, and possibly the glass. He wouldn't expect to find clots or pools of unclotted blood in this situation. A square of the upholstery would probably be cut out and used for analysis.

He would be able to perform a DNA match since the stain would provide all the DNA he needed. The salt water wouldn't change this result.

There are two things the M.E. might find amiss that could raise his level of suspicion. One would be the bloodstain pattern. If it looked staged rather than the expected pattern in such an accident, he might question the scene. Another red flag would be an elevation of the anticoagulant EDTA in the blood, but only if he tested for it. EDTA is sometimes sprayed on vegetables in the grocery store to prolong their freshness, so we all have a trace amount in our blood. That means it would be very difficult to state that any level found in the victim was elevated. There is no normal level for comparison. Still, an excessive concentration might give him pause and give you a nice thread to follow through your story.

Would Glycerol Used as a Blood Preservative Likely Be Found in Blood Used to Stage a Crime Scene?

Q: In my story someone tampers with a crime scene by planting blood evidence from a bag of blood preserved with glycerol and then frozen. My questions are these:

Does the M.E. routinely check blood obtained at a crime scene for evidence of previous freezing?

Would freezing hamper DNA typing?

If the blood was thawed by an amateur rather than being properly handled, would the blood have a similar appearance to fresh blood and would the presence of glycerol still be detectable even if it was not specifically being sought?

If a test was made on the sample for illegal narcotics, would the presence of glycerol be detected?

A: Blood at a crime scene is usually collected with cotton swabs, which are stored in glass vials until testing. Though microscopic examination of a liquid sample of blood might yield evidence that the blood had been frozen (ice crystal fragmentation of the red blood cells), this is not routinely done and couldn't be done from the blood collected on a swab.

DNA testing doesn't rely on intact cells, so freezing and thawing, clotting, or drying of the blood would have no effect on DNA matching.

The thawed blood, if spread around the floor or on furniture or bedsheets, would look like blood from any other source. Of course, the absence of clotting might suggest that the blood had some type of anticoagulant such as EDTA or glycerol added. This depends on how quickly the crime scene is discovered. If found immediately, any pools of blood would develop clots fairly quickly (in a matter of minutes) rather than stay liquid. If found later, these pools of blood will have clotted and will have a jellylike consistency. If they didn't clot, the M.E. would suspect the presence of an anticoagulant. If it is found even later, after the blood has dried, the M.E.'s task of determining whether the blood had clotted before drying would be difficult if not impossible.

Glycerol is an organic alcohol that has many industrial uses. It is the basic ingredient of the gums and resins used in exterior house paint and other protective coatings. It is used as an emulsifier and stabilizer in ice cream, shortening, and baked goods. It is used in the production of nitroglycerin. And relevant to your question, it is used as a protective medium for the freezing of red blood cells (to prevent the ice crystal fragmentation of the cells), sperm cells, corneas, and other living tissues.

Of course, if the M.E. tested for glycerol, he would find it, but that isn't necessarily part of a routine drug screen. Different labs have different protocols for what they test and what they don't. This means that if it fits your story to have the glycerol not found, or vice versa, it'll work.

How Soon Do Strangulation Bruises Appear?

Q: If a person tries to strangle another, how soon would visible marks occur on the neck? What would be their nature? Would the pressure indicate whether the person was right- or left-handed?

A: The marks are basically contusions or bruises, just like those acquired when you run into a door or table. The bruising appears in a very few minutes. The seepage of blood into the tissues from damaged capillary blood vessels causes the bluish discolorations. If a victim is strangled to death, the heart stops beating, and the blood in the vessels clots fairly quickly. Once the blood has clotted, bruising is no longer possible. In other words, strangling a dead person will not leave bruises.

The bruises appear from the blood that seeps out during the strangulation, before death. It happens almost immediately, though the surface discolorations we associate with contusions may take several minutes to appear.

The typical strangulation marks are the same bluish discolorations around the neck. These marks often are very distinctive and may outline the fingers or, if it is a ligature-type strangulation, even reveal the pattern of the rope, chain, or whatever was used.

The more pressure, the more bruising. A right-handed person tends to have a stronger right hand, and vice versa for a lefty, so the M.E. might be able to determine handedness of the killer from the bruises. At least he might be able to make an educated guess, which is what a great deal of forensics is about anyway.

When Does a Decomposing Body Begin to Smell?

Q: All things being equal, roughly how long would it take for an undiscovered dead body in a home begin to smell strongly enough to attract the attention of neighbors?

A: In general, twenty-four to forty-eight hours. That's when the body would start to get ripe, and things would get worse from there.

Decomposition of dead bodies is due to two different processes. Autolysis is the aseptic (without bacteria) breakdown of the body's cells and tissues. It is due to the action of the enzymes that normally exist within the cells—sort of a "self-digestion." These are chemical reactions, and they are accelerated by heat and slowed by cold.

The second is putrefaction, which is bacterially mediated. The bacteria that cause this process come both from the environment and from the normal bacteria that reside in the corpse's colon. These bacteria, like the above-mentioned intracellular enzymes, prefer a warm and cozy environment. So putrefaction is also accelerated by a higher ambient temperature and slowed in a colder environment.

In your situation the corpse would begin to smell in roughly twenty-four hours or less in a bedroom in New Orleans in August; a week or longer in an unheated apartment in Chicago in January. In a more temperate climate, a day or two should do it.

Do the M.E. and Police Use Vicks VapoRub to Mask the Odor of Decomposing Bodies?

Q: What is the substance that many coroners place on their upper lip when visiting a crime scene or performing an autopsy (presumably to offset the smell)? Does it have special properties, and, if so, can other substances (such as Vicks VapoRub) be used when it isn't available?

A: Yes, Vicks VapoRub is often used. Also, a surgical mask sprinkled with a peppermint concentrate is used by surgeons who must debride (the removal of dead and/or infected tissues) malodorous wounds such as those infected with gas gangrene (clostridia). Trust me, the smell of this is absolutely the worst thing you can encounter. It will literally knot your stomach and make your eyes water. The peppermint helps marginally. If the debridement is extensive and takes some time to accomplish, several surgeons may work in rotation so they can spell each other every twenty minutes or so because the odor of gas gangrene is that oppressive.

When the police or the crime scene technicians must work near a decomposing corpse, they often swipe a bit of VapoRub on their upper lip to mask the smell.

Fortunately, our olfactory nerve (the nerve that connects the odor-sensing cells in the nose to the brain) fatigues quickly. This means its ability to transmit smell signals to the brain weakens as exposure to the odor continues, and thus the intensity of the odor declines. Everyone has experienced this. After a very few minutes a noxious odor becomes more tolerable, and a faint odor fades and may disappear altogether. Even the wonderful aroma of warm apple pie is most intense when first detected.

Does a Cold Room Delay Detection of the Odor of Body Decomposition?

Q: My scenario is as follows: A mystery writer comes home from a luncheon, has a nap, writes until bedtime, goes to bed, gets up the next morning, and works until lunch-

time, when the police arrive at the door. They are looking for her husband (a cop), with whom she hasn't lived
for seven months; he didn't show up for duty the night
before. The officers discover him dead in the den. The
door was closed, and the air-conditioning has been on.
These are my questions: Would the smell of the decomposing body be prevalent in the house after twenty-four
to thirty-six hours? Is it plausible that the writer wouldn't
know that the corpse is in the closed-off room?

A: The short answer is yes.

Body decomposition begins immediately after death. Bacteria,
both external and those that live within the intestine, go to work
on the tissues, and under normal circumstances the smell of rotting
flesh is apparent in twenty-four to forty-eight hours. This timeline
depends on many things, particularly the ambient temperature. A
warm environment quickens bacterial growth and thus the process
of decomposition (like an incubator), while a colder one slows it
(like a refrigerator).

If the room is warm, the odor of decomposition may appear in
twenty-four hours or less; if cool, due to a low outside temperature
or from air-conditioning, it may take three or four days or more. In
this case your timing would work out. The AC would slow the
process, and the closed door would help contain the odor.

How Long Does It Take for an Unburied Body to Skeletonize?

Q: My question is about a character who is killed and left
unburied in the elements during May in the mountains
of the Northwest. The area has had an early spring,
with warm days and cool nights. Along with the usual
animal population there are bears and big cats.

How much decomposition would take place in four
to five weeks? I know the bones would be scattered and
hair would still be present. Is it possible the bones
would be relatively clean in that amount of time?

A: The time required for skeletonization of a body varies greatly
and depends on many factors. In your scenario the factors that
would favor rapid loss of tissues would include the following:

The warm weather, which hastens bacterial-mediated decomposition
The body being unburied and exposed to the air, weather,
bacteria, and predators
The length of the exposure

It is likely that after four or five weeks only skeletal remains,
teeth, and hair would be found. And as you noted, some bones
might be missing altogether, and others could be spread over a
wide area as predators carried them away.

What Is Calor Mortis?

Q: What is calor mortis? The color of the body after
death? Does the body change color after death?

A: Calor mortis is a rarely used term that does indeed refer to the
postmortem color of the body.

At death, cardiac function ceases, and the blood stagnates and settles according to the dictates of gravity. This results in postmortem
lividity, which becomes fixed in six to eight hours. This is a bluish,
grayish, purplish discoloration of the tissues in the dependent areas.

The remainder of the body takes on a pale, waxy, or rubbery

appearance. The acral areas (toes, fingers, ears, and sometimes the lips) may retain a slight bluish hue. Occasionally, the entire body has a very faint bluish or even a yellowish tint.

The term "calor mortis," which I could find little reference to in the medical literature, seems to mean this overall change in color, not the areas of lividity for which the term "livor mortis" is sometimes used.

Under What Circumstances Is Body Mummification Likely to Occur?

Q: In the book I'm writing, someone finds the mummified remains of a child who had disappeared ten years earlier. Where would be the best place for the body to be discovered so that the mummification would be realistic?

A: The preservation of an intact body can occur under varying circumstances. Freezing, in areas of permafrost, has preserved bodies for hundreds and even thousands of years. The same can be said for peat bogs. A bog is a wet, spongy, typically low-lying area that is composed chiefly of peat and sphagnum moss. It is typically acidic, and bodies that have sunk into the bog are spared bacterial degradation and may be well preserved when discovered years later.

But true mummification requires a dry climate. It can be either cold or warm, but it must be dry, preferably though not necessarily with a moving air current. It is desiccation (drying out or dehydration) of the body that leads to mummy formation. Also, the lack of moisture does not favor bacterial growth so that decomposition is halted or slowed.

As the corpse dries out, the muscles, organs, and skin shrink and become dark brown or black and leathery in quality. Depending on environmental conditions, this process may take several weeks or months. Once established, the mummified corpse can remain intact for years or decades.

As far as location of the corpse is concerned, any place that is dry, sheltered from the weather, and protected from predators would work. An attic, basement, or crawl space in a house or other structure can supply the right conditions. Desert burial can also.

Another possibility for long-term preservation of a body is adipocere formation. Adipocere is a waxy substance derived from body fat, and it was first described by Antoine Fourcroy in 1789.

The formation of adipocere is an alternative to complete putrefaction of the body. In reality, both putrefaction and adipocere formation begin in most corpses. If environmental factors favor bacterial growth and thus putrefaction, the body will deteriorate; if they inhibit bacterial growth and favor adipocere formation, the body will be preserved. In some cases the corpse does both so that part of the body is preserved and part is destroyed.

Adipocere formation requires certain conditions. If the body is buried in damp soil, immersed in water, or placed in a crypt or vault, adipocere can result. The key here is that moisture is required. Under these circumstances the anaerobic (meaning it doesn't require oxygen to grow) bacterium *clostridia perfringens* (the same culprit that produces gas gangrene) goes to work on the body, producing lecithinase, an enzyme that causes hydrolysis and hydrogenation of the corpse's fat. The result of this action is the formation of adipocere.

Adipocere is a waxy substance that varies in color from white to pinkish to gray or greenish gray. It takes three to twelve months to form and may last for decades, though it tends to become more brittle as the years pass.

The importance of this process is that instead of the usual dissolution of the tissues by the putrefaction process, the formation of adipocere casts the body permanently in its postmortem shape.

Some facial features and knife or bullet wounds may be well pre-served. Basically, the corpse looks like a wax doll.

Either of these types of mummification should fit your needs.

Is It Possible to Obtain Fingerprints from a Mummified Corpse?

Q: Can fingerprints be obtained from mummified remains?

A: Sometimes. It depends, of course, on the degree of deteriora-tion that the body has undergone. Typically, in well-preserved mummified corpses, the fingers are dark, shriveled, and leathery. Soaking them in a 20 percent acetic acid (the acid found in vine-gar) solution for twenty-four to forty-eight hours may swell them to normal size and reveal the finger pad ridges. Glycerin has been used for the same purpose. One novel method that has worked is to cut away the skin of the finger pad and press it flat with a level or cylindrical metal object. This may also expose the ridges.

Does a Body Mummify If It Has Been Bricked into a Wall for Several Years?

Q: What would the corpse of an average-sized young woman look like after being bricked up in an alcove of a house for several years? The space is in the interior of the house and is dry and has no openings (although, of course, no space is truly airtight). The house is in the Lake District of England, it's unoccupied, and it is nei-ther cooled in summer nor heated in winter. Would the body mummify, or would all parts except the skeleton decompose? When a body mummifies, do the eyeballs dry out, shrink, and sink back into the sockets?

A: Either mummification or skeletalization could happen. If the ambient air is humid, such as near the seacoast, skeletalization would likely occur. The humidity would favor bacterial growth and putrefaction of the tissues. But if the air is dry, most likely the body would mummify. The skin would desiccate (dry out), become dark brown or black, take on a leathery consistency, and shrink onto the skeleton as the muscles and internal organs also desiccated—like shrink-wrap. The entire corpse would appear small, and the arms and legs would likely contract into a fetal position if the space allowed.

Yes, the eyeballs would shrink down to nothing or perhaps a pea-sized hard knot that wouldn't be readily visible. The eye sockets would appear empty or caved in.

While either could occur, a mummified body is much more visual and spooky.

Will a Body Encased in Concrete Mummify?

Q: I want a victim's body to be found four years after his death by gunshot wound. Right now I have the body unearthed when a fire destroys a building whose foundation was laid four years earlier. The building burns down to the foundation, and the body is found while workers are clearing the lot and digging up the remaining concrete. What state would the body be in at this point? Mummified? Could he be identified? Also, at the time of the murder, I haven't figured out how to get the body into the excavation prior to the concrete being poured without someone noticing.

A: The body could be either skeletonized or mummified. If the latter, it would likely look dark and leathery. Identification might depend on dental records and possibly fingerprints. There are techniques for recovering prints from mummified remains.

The bullet could be within the mummy or nearby even if skeletonized. Maybe a fractured or nicked rib or other bone plus a bullet fragment would be the tipoff and lead the M.E. to determine that a gunshot was the cause of death.

If the body is buried beneath concrete, mummification becomes more likely since less oxygen would reach the body, and decomposition would thus be slowed or halted. Also, animal predation and the effects of weather would be absent.

Depending on the size and depth of the excavation, the body could be partially buried (actually, a simple soil covering would suffice), and those working the cement truck wouldn't notice a slight bump in the floor of the trench dug for the foundation.

Is It Possible to Trick a Lie Detector?

Q: In my story I want the murderer to undergo a lie detector test and pass it even though he is guilty. Is it possible to trick a lie detector machine? If so, how?

A: A lie detector (polygraph) examination is not an exact test, and for this reason it is not typically admissible in court. Law enforcement uses it primarily to narrow the focus of their investigation by excluding some suspects. Though not completely accurate in this regard, it does help at times.

The polygraph ("poly" means many; "graph" means to write) tests several of the body's responses to stress. It consists of a blood pressure cuff, a chest band to measure respiration, a skin electrode that measures the galvanic (electrical) skin response, and a recording device to collect the data. Under stress the blood pressure and heart rate increase, as does the depth and frequency of respiration, and sweat leaks from the pores. The electrolytes (sodium, potassium, and chloride) in sweat increase the electrical conductivity of the skin. This is called the galvanic response. The examiner looks for stress-induced increases in each of these parameters as a clue to likely deception.

During the pretest interview, the examiner asks questions to determine if the individual has any illnesses or psychiatric disorders or is taking any medications that might interfere with these responses and thus invalidate the test.

The easiest way to defeat the test is to make it inconclusive—that is, one in which the examiner is unable to discern if deception is present or not. People who are histrionic or subject to extreme nervousness or panic attacks are difficult if not impossible to examine. Faking a histrionic reaction may invalidate or confuse the results.

During the test the examiner asks some questions that are low stress and easy to answer truthfully: Did you have eggs for breakfast this morning? Do you live at 123 Elm Street? Simple and nonstressful. He intersperses questions that are more stressful or more directly related to the crime in question: Did you have a confrontation with Mr. Jones? Were you at his home on the evening of June 3? Did you kill Mr. Jones with a hammer? A truthful person will react the same to these questions, while the guilty party will become stressed when answering the pointed questions. A high-strung individual might react regardless of the benignity of the question. He would panic at everything so that his blood pressure, heart rate, respiration, and galvanic skin response jump if someone says, "Boo."

Forcing a panic-like response to every question could cloud the deception and make the test inclusive. The killer could purposefully tighten his muscles, breathe more deeply than usual, concentrate on anything stressful, even his own guilt, regardless of the question, or even put a tack in his shoe to step on after each question. The examiner might not be able to tell the difference between these forced stresses and the real stress of lying.

The other option would be to go the other way—that is, remain calm throughout. Some sociopaths simply don't feel guilt the way normal people do. Though not common, they may be naturally able to defeat the test because they don't *feel* guilty. Or your perp might employ certain relaxation techniques to blunt the stress responses. Biofeedback, imagery, breath control, and other meditative techniques might work. Or he could use drugs. Alcohol, narcotics, and other sedative substances might help if he can act sober enough to take the test in the first place.

Another choice might be the group of drugs we call beta-blockers. Common ones are Inderal, Tenormin, and Lopressor. Taking 10 milligrams (mg) of Inderal or 25 to 50 mg of Tenormin or 50 mg of Lopressor an hour or two before the test might do the trick. These drugs block the effect of adrenaline on the cardiovascular system. They decrease the blood pressure and slow the heart rate. They also have a calming effect on the brain and may lessen stress-induced sweating. Thus, they might blunt the stress responses enough for the perp to "pass" the test.

Can an Intoxicated Person Fake a Field Sobriety Test?

Q: My character is intoxicated when he must rush to the rescue of a loved one. His speeding car is stopped by the police. It's a long story, but there is no way he can explain his situation to the police in any believable fashion. Is it possible he could fake a field sobriety test or a Breathalyzer or blood test for alcohol intoxication?

A: Tricking a Breathalyzer or a blood alcohol test is virtually impossible. They are accurate, and you can't hide the alcohol in your bloodstream or on your exhaled breath.

Passing a field sobriety test while intoxicated is very difficult. The reason for this is that alcohol affects the cerebellum of the brain, which controls balance, gait, movement, and coordination. The field tests are designed to evaluate cerebellar function, which in the presence of alcohol is abnormal.

Standing with your eyes closed, arms spread to the side, or on one foot leads to swaying and perhaps falling. Walking a straight line, heel to toe, becomes a wavering, wandering stroll. Touching your finger to your nose results in poking your eye. And looking to the side while facing straight ahead causes the eyes to bounce laterally. (This is called nystagmus.) Regardless of how hard you concentrate on these tasks, the alcohol-soaked cerebellum will prevent performance in a normal fashion. Book him, Dano.

Can Fingerprints Be Lifted from Human Skin?

Q: Can fingerprints be lifted from human skin—for example, from the neck of a victim who was manually strangled? How long after death do the prints remain detectable?

A: The short answer is yes, but the window of opportunity is very short. It depends on many factors, but prints have been lifted from skin and used in identifying perps. On living flesh they last about sixty to ninety minutes. On corpses it is a little longer, depending on environmental conditions. The sooner the prints are collected, the better.

There are several techniques for lifting prints from skin.

The Kromekote Technique: A Kromekote card is pressed over the suspected print (unexposed Polaroid film may also be used), and then it is dusted with black print powder to expose the print. The print is then photographed and finally lifted with cellophane tape.

The Magna-Brush Technique: The body or body part is brushed with MacDonnell Magna Jet Black Powder (which is actually extremely fine iron filings), and any prints that appear are photographed. Typically, a light is directed toward the print from whatever angle exposes the ridge details best.

Electron Emission Radiography: The skin where the suspected print is located is dusted with a fine lead powder and then examined by X ray. The bulky size of the X ray equipment limits the usefulness of this technique, however.

Iodine-Silver-Plate Technique: The suspected area is exposed to an iodine vapor, which is absorbed by the moisture in the latent print. It is then dusted with a silver powder that reacts with the iodine to form silver iodide. This compound darkens when exposed to intense light (silver iodide is a component of photographic film), and the print becomes visible. Alternatively, the iodine fuming may be followed by an application of alpha-naphthoflavone to reveal the ridge pattern.

Cyanoacrylate Fuming: After the application of this substance, the latent print appears white, which may be difficult to see and photograph on light skin. To make it more visible, the fumed prints are colored with various biologic stains, commercial dyes, or TEC (Europium ThenoylTrifluoroAcetone ortho-phenanthroline or EuTTAPhen or simply Europium complex, for short). The result is best viewed under an alternative light source such as an ultraviolet light.

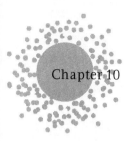

Chapter 10

THE CORONER, THE CRIME LAB,
AND THE AUTOPSY

Who Can Serve as Coroner?

Q: My story is set in a small town. For plot purposes the county coroner (or is it the medical examiner?) is also the local sheriff. Can this happen? Who can serve as coroner? What are his or her qualifications?

A: Yes, the sheriff can be the coroner, but he cannot be the medical examiner. Let me explain.

There is often a great deal of confusion regarding the roles of the coroner and the medical examiner (M.E.). The coroner is an elected official. He is responsible for all the legal aspects of death: death certificates, court appearances, and overseeing all the functions of the coroner's office. The M.E., by definition, is a physician who specializes in forensics and is usually a forensic pathologist.

Often, the elected coroner is the M.E., and there is a move in most states to require M.E. credentials for anyone running for the position of coroner. In jurisdictions where the coroner is not required to be medically trained, an M.E. is appointed who has the proper training to perform the forensic duties needed. He is often called the deputy coroner.

In most metropolitan areas of the United States the M.E. is the coroner. However, if your story is set in a small remote town, the coroner could be the local sheriff, undertaker, or auto mechanic. Here, the possibilities are wide open and the story twists endless.

When Are Autopsies Done, and Who Can Request Them?

Q: Under what circumstances are autopsies required? Who officially makes the request? Can the family of the victim prevent an autopsy?

A: The laws that govern the coroner's or medical examiner's office vary in different jurisdictions. However, most operate under similar guidelines. Violent deaths (accidents, homicides, suicides); those that occur at the workplace; those that are suspicious, sudden, or unexpected; those that occur while the person is incarcerated; and those that occur within twenty-four hours of admission to a hospital would typically become "coroner's cases."

Physicians are often asked to sign a death certificate for a patient they know who has died at home. If the patient had severe heart disease or cancer or any disease where death is likely, the physician usually signs the certificate, and the coroner isn't typically involved.

If a patient enters a hospital and dies from any cause within the first twenty-four hours, it automatically becomes a coroner's case. The twenty-four hours is extended indefinitely in the case of a patient who enters the hospital unconscious and never regains consciousness prior to death. The coroner may then contact the physician caring for the patient, and if a satisfactory reason is apparent, the coroner signs the death certificate, and that's the end of it. If the death is unusual or unexplained, an autopsy will take place.

In addition, a court may request an autopsy, as can the coroner, in any case where one might be helpful. The coroner has subpoena power for records and testimony, and has jurisdiction over the body in such cases.

No, in most jurisdictions the family cannot prevent an autopsy by refusing permission. No permission is required if the medical examiner or coroner or the court deems that an autopsy is needed. However, since our legal system allows lawsuits for almost anything, the family could perhaps file suit to block the procedure, in which case a judge would decide the matter. Most likely the autopsy would be performed.

How Detailed Are Routine Autopsies?

Q: How detailed are most autopsies in situations in which the dead person would not at first blush appear to be the victim of foul play? I'm thinking of plot situations, for instance, in which a wife is poisoned or drowned by a seemingly loving husband and the circumstances appear accidental or otherwise not suspicious.

A: The key issue for the killer in this type of circumstance is to prevent an autopsy in the first place. If the victim is elderly, chronically ill with potentially lethal diseases such as heart or lung disease, diabetes, or cancer, and is under the care of a physician, the physician may sign the death certificate stating that the death was due to one of these processes. The certificate would be filed with the coroner's office, of course, but more than likely it would not make him sit up, take notice, and ask questions. The murder would go undiscovered. On the other hand, if the victim was a teenager, both the physician and the coroner would probably be suspicious, and an autopsy would be requested.

Even routine autopsies are typically very thorough. A gross exam and dissection is followed by microscopic tissue examinations and toxicologic studies. The coroner then issues a "cause of death." That said, a "medico-legal autopsy"—that is, one in which the cause of death is suspicious or unexplained—is even more thorough and is generally performed by a pathologist trained in forensics. In your scenario the medical examiner could easily determine that the cause of death was a poison or drowning. As for who pushed her in the water or gave her the poison, your sleuth will have to figure that out.

What Information Does an Autopsy Report Contain?

Q: What information is contained in the typical autopsy report? Does the coroner or medical examiner always state the cause of death?

A: Each pathologist has his or her own way of preparing an autopsy report, but certain things must be addressed for the report to be complete. And yes, one of those is the cause of death as well as a determination as to whether the death was natural or possibly criminal.

The name, age, sex, and race of the deceased, the estimated time of death, the location of death or where the body was discovered, and the date and time of the autopsy examination are commonly indicated on the first page. Also included are the name and qualifications of the person performing the exam, the names of all persons present, and a brief note concerning the circumstances of the death.

The first section of the actual examination would be titled "External Examination." The M.E. would describe the appearance of the body and comment on any abnormalities, including external injuries and signs of medical intervention. For example, if the person died in a hospital, he may have IV needles and various tubes in place. These are not removed by hospital personnel before the body is sent to the coroner's office since they may be valuable evidence in cases of homicide or medical malpractice. Any injuries from trauma, gunshots, or knives, or external marks of any kind, including tattoos, surgical scars, old wound scars, cutaneous (skin) diseases, and birthmarks, would be commented on and photographed.

The next section would be titled "Internal Examination" and would deal with what the M.E. found inside the body. This section is typically subdivided into these areas: head, neck, body cavities, cardiovascular system (heart and blood vessels), respiratory system (nose, throat, larynx, trachea, bronchial tubes, lungs), gastrointestinal system (esophagus, stomach, intestines), hepatobiliary system (liver, gallbladder, pancreas), genitourinary system (kidneys, bladder, prostate, ovaries, uterus), endocrine system (thyroid, pituitary, and adrenal glands), lymphoreticular system (spleen, lymph nodes), musculoskeletal system (bones, muscles), and central nervous system (brain, spinal cord). Under each of these headings the M.E. would describe the gross and microscopic appearance of the relevant organs and tissues as well as any abnormalities found.

Next would come a summary of the pertinent and relevant findings. As an example, the summary of the exam on someone who died of a heart attack might include the following:

1. Cardiovascular System
   A. Extensive atherosclerotic vascular disease involving the left main, left anterior descending, and circumflex coronary arteries
   B. Large area of myocardial necrosis in the distribution of the left anterior descending coronary artery

This means the person had severe hardening of the arteries and died from a heart attack (myocardial necrosis).

Last would be a statement titled "Conclusion." Here the M.E. would state his belief as to the cause of death and whether the death was natural or at the hand of another. He would then sign the report, making it official.

Attachments to the report would detail any toxicologic, ballistic,

DNA, or other examinations that had been performed in that particular case.

What Information Is Placed in a Death Certificate, and Who Can Sign It?

Q: I have a few questions regarding death certificates. Who can sign a death certificate? Is one completed for everyone who dies? I'm also confused by the terms "mode," "cause," and "manner" of death. Are they all the same thing? What information is placed on the actual certificate?

A: In most if not all jurisdictions a death certificate must be signed by a licensed physician. If someone dies in the hospital or from an expected death (someone with terminal cancer or heart disease, for example) at home, his or her personal or treating physician will likely sign the certificate. If not, the M.E. or coroner will. Of course, if the death is under suspicious circumstances, unexpected, unusual, or occurs within twenty-four hours of a hospital admission, the coroner would be involved, and he would sign the certificate whether an autopsy was performed or not.

Everyone who dies should have a legally registered death certificate.

Regarding the terms you mentioned, you are not the only one who finds them confusing. Simply put, the "mode of death" refers to the pathophysiologic abnormality that led to death—for example, a cardiac arrest. The "cause of death" is what led to this abnormality, such as a gunshot wound to the heart. The "manner of death" is a legal, not a medical, statement and refers to whether the death was natural, a homicide, a suicide, or an accident.

The certificate contains the usual demographic information: name, address, age, sex, race, occupation, place of death (if known), and information regarding the next of kin. The physician then adds the immediate cause of death (actually, this is often a combination of cause and mode—see, it is confusing) as well as conditions that led to or contributed to the stated cause and the duration that each of these was probably present. For example, in someone with high blood pressure and diabetes who suddenly fell dead from a heart attack, the physician might state the cause as follows:

Cause of Death	Duration
Immediate Cause: Cardiac Arrest	Immediate
Due To: Acute Myocardial Infarction	Minutes
Due To: Atherosclerotic Cardiovascular Disease	Years
Contributing Conditions: Diabetes, Hypertension	

He then signs and dates the certificate, making it official.

How Is the Time of Death Determined?

Q: How does the coroner determine the time of death?

A: Unless the death is witnessed, it is impossible to determine the exact time of death. The medical examiner can only estimate the time of demise. It is important to note that this estimated time can vary greatly from the legal time of death, which is the time recorded on the death certificate, and the physiologic time of death, which is when vital functions actually ceased.

The legal time of death is when the body was discovered or the time a doctor or other qualified person pronounced the victim dead. These may differ by days, weeks, or even months if the body is not found until well after physiologic death has occurred. For example, if a serial killer kills a victim in July but the body is not discovered until October, the physiologic death took place in July, but the legal death is marked as October.

That said, the coroner can estimate the physiologic time of death with some degree of accuracy. He uses the changes that occur in the human body after death to help him in this endeavor. These changes consist of measuring the drop in body temperature, the degree of rigidity (rigor mortis), the degree of discoloration (livor mortis or lividity), the stage of body decomposition, and other factors.

Body temperature drops approximately 1.5 degrees per hour after death until it reaches the temperature of the environment. Obviously, this measure is greatly affected by the ambient temperature. A body in the snow in Minnesota in January and one in a Louisiana swamp in August will lose heat at widely divergent rates. These factors must be considered in any estimate of time of death.

Rigor mortis typically follows a predictable pattern. Rigidity begins in the small muscles of the face and neck and progresses downward to the larger muscles. This process of progressive rigidity takes about twelve hours. Then the process reverses itself, with rigidity being lost in the same fashion, beginning with the small muscles and progressing to the larger muscles. This phase takes another twelve to thirty-six hours. So rigor is useful only in the first forty-eight hours. After that the corpse is flaccid (limp), and the M.E. cannot determine if death occurred forty-eight or more hours earlier using this criterion alone.

The reason for the rigidity is the loss of adenosine triphosphate, or ATP, from the muscles. ATP is the compound that serves as energy for muscular activity, and its presence and stability depend on a steady supply of oxygen and nutrients, which are lost with the cessation of cardiac activity. As the supply of stable ATP declines, the muscles tend to contract, which produces the rigidity. The later loss of rigidity and the appearance of flaccidity (relaxation) of the muscles occur when the muscle tissue itself begins to break down.

As decomposition and putrefaction occur, the contractile components (the actin and myosin filaments within the muscles that are responsible for muscular contraction) decay, and the muscle loses its contractile properties and relaxes.

Lividity is caused by stagnation of blood in the vessels. It lends a purplish color to the tissues. The blood, following the dictates of gravity, seeps into the dependent parts of the body—along the back and buttocks of a victim who is supine after death. Initially, this discoloration can be shifted by rolling the body to a different position, but by six to eight hours it becomes fixed. If a body is found facedown but with fixed lividity along the back, then the body was moved at least six hours after death, but not earlier than three or four, or the lividity would have shifted to the newly dependent area.

At death the body begins to decompose. Bacteria begin to work on the tissues, and depending on ambient conditions, by twenty-four to forty-eight hours the smell of rotting flesh appears and the skin takes on a progressive greenish red color. By three days gas forms in the body cavities and beneath the skin, which may leak fluid and split. From there things get worse. Add to this the predation by animals and insects, and the body can become completely skeletonized before long. In hot, humid climes this can happen in three or four weeks, sometimes less.

As you can see, this is a very inexact science and is greatly altered by the environment. In cold areas body temperature changes are magnified, but decomposition changes are slowed. The inverse is true for hot, humid climes.

Would Storing a Body in a Cold Room Hinder the Determination of Cause of Death?

Q: Is there a way that my character could try to cover up a crime of passion by cooling the body (in a wine room, perhaps) and then moving it but wind up with a pool of blood when the corpse heats up in its new location? The crime occurs in the hot Arizona summer, if that makes a difference.

A: Actually, cooling the body would work against the killer by preserving the evidence. This is exactly what the coroner does when he stores a body in a refrigerated room until the autopsy can be performed. Cooling slows the process of decomposition and putrefaction. Gunshot wounds, knife wounds, and any poisons would be preserved longer and would make the coroner's job easier.

On the other hand, if the body was left outdoors in the heat, bacterial putrefaction would be greatly accelerated, so that by the time the body was discovered, tissue decomposition may be so far advanced that gun and knife wounds would be difficult to evaluate—that is, the depth and width of stab wounds and the characteristics of gunshot wounds that help determine how close the gun was to the victim, and so forth, would be lost in severely degraded tissues. If the decay was far advanced, even some poisons may no longer be detectable.

As for leaving a blood pool later, I'm afraid that won't work. Bleeding or oozing of blood requires that the heart still be pumping and the blood still circulating, which means that bleeding ceases at death. In fact, at death all the blood in the body clots very quickly, in a matter of minutes, and thus couldn't flow or ooze or drip and form a pool outside the body. Unlike ice cream, blood doesn't melt. Once it's clotted, it can't unclot.

This was brilliantly and subtly illustrated in the Coen brothers' 1984 film noir classic *Blood Simple*. The husband is shot as he sits behind his desk and is presumed dead. Later, another character comes in and sees the "corpse." The camera angles on the victim's hand, dangling above a pool of blood, and we see blood ooze down his fingers. At that moment the knowledgeable observer says, "Aha! He's not dead." Less clever viewers have to wait another scene or two to learn the same thing.

Can the Coroner Distinguish Between Electrocution and a Heart Attack as the Cause of Death?

Q: My victim is electrocuted while sailing by touching a boarding ladder that has been electrified, causing an apparent heart attack. Would there be any physical signs at autopsy that might show the victim died as a result of the electrocution rather than a heart attack? Skin surface burns, and so forth?

A: The autopsy findings depend on the amount of voltage applied. If the voltage was high, burn marks would be left at the points of contact and grounding—that is, the entry and exit points of the current. These would be readily identifiable by the medical examiner. Also, when a strong electrical current flows through the body, it damages (cooks) everything in its path, and these effects can be seen when the various tissues are examined microscopically. This is particularly true of the liver, which seems to be prone to this type of injury.

If the voltage was low, no skin changes would occur. And to be puristic, in this situation the victim wouldn't die from a heart attack (myocardial infarction, or MI). In its true and simplest definition an MI means that a coronary artery (the arteries that course over the surface of the heart and supply blood to the heart muscle) became blocked, and a portion of the heart dies due to lack of blood supply. In a true MI the M.E. would find the blocked artery and the damage to the heart muscle. An electric current could not directly cause this.

Though a lower-voltage electrical shock would not cause heart muscle damage, it could precipitate a lethal change in heart rhythm, such as ventricular tachycardia or ventricular fibrillation. These could only be diagnosed if an electrocardiogram (EKG) was connected to the victim at the time the arrhythmias occurred. This is unlikely in the case you present.

At autopsy the heart would likely appear normal in this circumstance, so the electric shock would not be detectable. With no MI and no skin burns, the M.E. would probably assume the victim died of a cardiac arrhythmia, which, of course, is exactly what happened.

As you would expect, a voltage between these two would yield mixed results.

Can the M.E. Distinguish Between Blunt Trauma and Stab Wounds as the Cause of Death?

Q: My victim is a young female in the very early stages of pregnancy. The perp is furious about the baby and strikes her in the abdomen. My theory is that this would probably not be sufficient to induce a miscarriage but would definitely leave evidence for the M.E. Right?

Thrown off balance, the victim falls and strikes her head on the edge of the bathtub. Would there be any clue as to what surface specifically caused the injury? Even without an indication of what caused the head injury, would there be some indication that this injury occurred prior to the fatal wounds? For plot purposes I'd like the unconscious victim to be moved elsewhere as a diversion, where multiple stab wounds would be inflicted as the ultimate cause of death.

The murder occurs on a summer night in Arizona, and the body is not discovered until the next day. Would the M.E. be able to determine the true cause of death?

A: The blow to the abdomen could or could not cause a miscarriage. If the force was strong enough and applied directly to the lower abdomen, it could damage the fetus, the placenta, or the uterus severely enough that the fetus would no longer be viable and a miscarriage would result. Or the blow could simply contuse (bruise) the abdominal wall. Your call, since either is possible.

The M.E. would likely see the contusion, unless the victim was killed only a few minutes after the blow. Bruises take a few minutes to appear. He would be able to tell that the blow was applied antemortem (before death) by the gross and microscopic nature of the contusion. Bruising results from a leakage of blood from injured microscopic capillaries and requires that blood flow, and therefore life, be present. After death the blood clots in a few minutes so that this leakage no longer occurs. Postmortem (after death) blows would not produce bruising.

The fall against the tub could be lethal or merely knock her unconscious (a concussion), as you proposed. The M.E. would be able to tell that this injury also was antemortem, and he might be able to ascertain the general shape of the object. Bathtub edge? Baseball bat? Metal pipe? Unless the enamel coating of the tub cracked and small pieces clung to her hair or skin, he probably wouldn't be able to go beyond guessing the general shape of the object.

One day in the desert wouldn't destroy much of the forensic evidence unless predators dismantled, consumed, and scattered the body. The M.E. would be able to determine that the cause of death was multiple stab wounds and that the other injuries were antemortem but not the proximate cause of death. He could, of course, determine that she was pregnant. And if a miscarriage occurred at the time of the beating, he would be able to determine that also.

Can the Coroner Distinguish Between Drug Overdose and Gunshot as the Cause of Death?

Q: Suppose a character is fatally shot (either by another party or by himself—to be determined) after ingesting

twenty-five tranquilizers. How would a medical examiner determine the time lapse between the ingestion of
the pills and the gunshot? Could he determine whether
the person was conscious and could shoot himself, as
opposed to being out cold, which would indicate homicide? What would the M.E. look for? What blood tests
or other tests would he run? How quickly can he get
results? If this occurred on a Friday night, what is the
soonest the autopsy would be done?

A: The time lapse between ingestion and death would be a best
guess. The data used by the M.E. in this circumstance would be
dissolved versus undissolved pills in the stomach, the presence of
other food materials, and the levels of the drug in the blood and
urine of the victim. Each drug has a known absorption rate and
excretion rate, but this is altered by other foods taken, other drugs
involved (either as part of the suicide/murder or medications that
the victim takes routinely), the age of the victim, what diseases the
victim has (particularly gastrointestinal problems), and a host of
other factors. Add to this that everyone is different, and the problem becomes more complex.

Digestion and absorption cease at death, so the stomach, blood,
and urine contents and their drug concentrations would be relatively frozen at that time. After analyses of these, the M.E. could
make a guess as to when the drug was taken. From the blood levels
he could also make a judgment as to the victim's physical and mental abilities. Each drug is different, of course, so the effects of the
particular drug used would be taken into account.

I know this is very general, but the problem is complex and
multifactorial. In your scenario you could go either way and be
okay. The M.E. could reach the conclusion that based on the stomach contents and blood levels, he believed the victim could not
have shot himself or he believed the exact opposite. Say the blood
levels of the drug were very high, at a level where the victim would

likely be in a coma; the M.E. would state that the death was a homicide. Or if the levels were low, he would state that the victim
could have pulled the trigger. Two different stories. The choice is
yours since either would work.

The testing of stomach, blood, and urine contents for drugs
could be done in a few hours if the drugs involved are common
and easily tested. If they are less common and require special testing, the samples may have to go to a more sophisticated lab, and
that could take weeks.

The autopsy would probably be done on Monday unless the
M.E. requested that it be done sooner; then it could be done
anytime.

Can the Coroner Determine the Cause of Death a Month Later?

Q: In my story, a male character is struck in the head with
a rock and left in a basement. This occurs during a cold
February in a northern climate. The nighttime temperatures are in the 20s, and there is snow on the ground.
Several days later the man is found dead, and the body is
moved to a remote area. A month later someone finds
the body and calls the police.

My questions: Is it more likely that the man was
killed by hitting his head on the rock or by later exposure? A month after death, can the coroner or M.E.
determine the cause of death and that the body was
moved?

A: The cause of death could be the blow to the head, or the
victim may merely have been rendered unconscious and then
froze to death—death from hypothermia. Though he may never
be completely sure, the M.E. would be able to make an educated

guess as to whether the blow was powerful enough to cause death. He would look for a fracture of the skull and, more important, signs of bleeding in and around the brain. We call these "intracranial bleeds," which basically is any bleed inside the cranium (skull). Bleeding within the brain itself is called an intracerebral bleed, and bleeding around the brain could be either a subdural or an epidural bleed, depending on exactly where the bleed occurs. Any of these can be deadly, especially if not treated fairly promptly. If the M.E. finds any of these at autopsy, he could reasonably conclude that the blow was the proximate cause of death. If he finds none of these, he might state that the cause of death was due to exposure and hypothermia.

At autopsy there may be no specific findings that indicate death from hypothermia. Alternatively, the characteristic brownish pink discoloration of the skin on the elbows, knees, and, less often, the face and flanks may be seen. The presence of these changes would support a finding that death occurred from freezing.

Since the weather you describe is cold, the body and these findings would likely be well preserved for a month or longer.

Lividity—the purplish discoloration of the skin due to settling of blood in the tissues after death—becomes fixed after six to eight hours. It settles in the dependent or lower areas of the body as dictated by gravity. Once it becomes fixed, moving the body will not result in a shift of the lividity to a newly dependent area. For example, if the victim dies while lying on his back, the lividity would settle along the back and buttocks. If he is rolled to his stomach several hours later, the fixed lividity does not shift but remains where it originally settled. If the lividity pattern doesn't match the body position at the time the corpse is discovered, then the M.E. would conclude that the body had been moved.

Is It Possible to Detect Morphine in a Body Two Months After Death?

Q: A woman kills her husband with IV morphine. She dresses him like a bum and dumps his body in an alley. He has never had dental work and never been finger-printed. Although the body is found soon after the murder, identification isn't made for two months.

Could the coroner find that the cause of death was morphine after this time period?

A: Yes. Morphine sulfate (MS) would remain in the tissues since all metabolic processes of the body shut down at death. Thus, the MS wouldn't be metabolized (broken down). Blood and tissue samples would likely show its presence.

This is particularly true in the circumstance you describe. Since the body was found soon after the murder, the remains would be well preserved, as would the forensic evidence. An autopsy would likely be performed fairly quickly to determine the cause of the unwitnessed death and to determine if the death was natural or possibly a homicide. The coroner would then store the body in a refrigerated environment until the identification was made.

If the body was found two months after death and was only skeletal remains, the M.E. would have a tougher time finding the MS.

Can a Blood Alcohol Level Be Determined in a "Floater" After Two Weeks?

Q: Is it possible for a body to float to the top in relatively cold water (about 55 degrees) after two weeks? Would it be possible, assuming that two-week period, for an autopsy to show the level of blood alcohol? Or would the alcohol dissipate?

A: "Floaters" are corpses found floating in a body of water. They present special problems for the M.E. in determining the time of death. Water temperature, of course, has an effect, as do local tides and predators. The general rule regarding decomposition is that one week on dry land equals two weeks for a submerged body.

To become a floater, a body must be in the water long enough for tissue decomposition from bacteria to begin. This process forms gas as a by-product, and the gas collects beneath the skin and in body cavities. Bodies tend to sink and then rise again in several days when the gas forms, adding buoyancy. They thus become floaters.

The M.E. should be able to determine the blood alcohol level since all metabolic processes cease at death. The level would be fairly stable until the body significantly decomposed. In your scenario the cold water would slow this process and preserve the alcohol longer. I think you would be on safe ground after two weeks at 55 degrees to allow your M.E. to make that determination.

How Long Does the Foam Around a Drowning Victim's Mouth Persist?

Q: My protagonist finds a floater out in the ocean. A gaseous foam is found around the victim's nose and mouth. The question is, how long does this foam last? An hour? Two? Also, my victim was shot in the abdomen, but she expired from drowning. The cause of death is not discovered until the autopsy is done. Am I crystal clear on that one?

A: The problem with your scenario is one of timing. A drowning victim may have frothy water coming from her mouth if she is pulled from the water fairly quickly—I'd guess within an hour or so. After that, perhaps blood-tinged water would leak from the mouth and nose, but it probably wouldn't be frothy since the lungs would have lost all their air and none would be left to "froth." Think ice cream soda; when the fizz is gone, it's just colored liquid. Froth requires air in the lungs, and in a drowning the air is expelled or absorbed into the water, and thus the lungs of someone who has been underwater for several hours are typically waterlogged.

In a floater, the body would have to be in the water for a while—long enough for tissue decomposition from bacteria to begin (see previous question). This process forms gas as a by-product, and the gas collects beneath the skin and in body cavities. Bodies tend to sink and then rise again in several days when the gas forms, adding buoyancy. They thus become floaters. Under these circumstances the hands and feet would swell (after several days), the outer layer of skin would separate from the underlying tissues (five to six days), the skin of the hands and the nails would separate (eight to ten days), the entire body would become swollen, and the tissues would become fragile and be easily damaged during removal from the water. But foaming from the mouth or nose would not be present.

Timing of the floating depends on several factors, including water temperature, currents, the size of the victim, and other variables. For example, a body will float after eight to ten days in warm water and two to three weeks in colder water. Cold slows the process of decomposition by slowing bacterial growth and, thus, gas formation.

So you have to decide which situation is best for you: a recent drowning where the victim is found underwater and dragged up and has foam around the mouth and nose, or a floater who pops up many days after the murder and does not have any foaming.

You are correct that an M.E. could determine the cause of death was drowning as opposed to the gunshot. He could also determine if it was a freshwater or a saltwater drowning. This is complex to explain, but an M.E. can tell the difference. (See the later question, "Can the Coroner Distinguish Between Freshwater and Saltwater Drowning?") This fact was used in the movie *Chinatown*.

From How Small a Sample Can DNA Be Obtained?

Q: I know that DNA samples can be obtained from blood, semen, tissue beneath a victim's fingernails, and other sources. My questions are these: How small a sample can be used? Can dried saliva or a strand of hair be used?

A: DNA resides in the nucleus of essentially every cell in the body and is unique to each of us. Notable exceptions are the red blood cells (RBCs) in the blood. Mature RBCs have no nuclei and thus no DNA. White blood cells (WBCs) do. When blood is used for DNA analysis, it is the DNA in WBCs that is tested.

Each person's DNA pattern is decided somewhat randomly at conception by which sperm fertilizes which egg. It is identical in every cell of an individual's body and remains unchanged throughout his or her lifetime. Thus, with the exception of identical twins, no two people have the same pattern. This is why DNA is so useful in determining if a given sample came from a particular person. Quite simply, if a match is made, the material could not have come from anyone else.

To extract DNA from a sample, the material must contain cells, though they do not have to be intact. That is, if you look at the sample under a microscope, there may be no intact cells visible, but DNA remains in the tissue or fluid residue. Thus, decomposed blood, semen, or body tissues can still yield usable samples. Even skeletal remains may have usable DNA in the marrow cavity or in the cells of the bone (osteocytes).

In regard to sample size, the larger, the better, but even traces of fluids or tissue can yield results. The polymerase chain reaction (PCR) method for DNA testing seems to work best for these small samples.

Saliva contains buccal cells (those that line the inside of the mouth), and the nuclei of these cells provide DNA for testing. Saliva can be gleaned from drinking glasses, bite marks, and postage stamps or envelopes. New techniques using fluorescence spectroscopy can identify very small areas of saliva residue on human skin. Saliva can sometimes be obtained from the face mask worn by an assailant during his attack or robbery. A case reported in *The Journal of Forensic Sciences* in 1999 illustrates how small a sample is needed for testing. The body of a female rape and murder victim was recovered from a river after five and a half hours had elapsed. A bite mark yielded enough saliva for DNA testing.

Hair contains no cells and therefore no DNA. But hair follicles do. Cut hair is unlikely to be useful for DNA analysis, but hair pulled from an assailant or shed by the attacker during the assault may be the "smoking gun" needed to convict him. A single hair follicle may provide enough DNA for testing.

Does the M.E. Use Tattoos and Body Marks for Corpse Identification?

Q: Does the coroner use distinctive body marks and tattoos to help identify unknown corpses? Would such marks be used if the hands and face of the victim had been destroyed or removed?

A: The coroner would use any and all means to ID a "John Doe."

Body marks such as tattoos or birthmarks are often helpful in suspect and corpse identification. They are often sketched or photographed as part of the booking process, although this is far from universal. If your suspect or corpse had body marks and if photos existed from a previous arrest, they could obviously be compared even if the photo was sent from another jurisdiction via e-mail or fax.

At autopsy the pathologist routinely photographs these as well as surgical and injury scars, particularly if a homicide is suspected.

Many tattoos and birthmarks are so distinctive as to be fairly strong ID evidence. In the case of a corpse, a previous cell mate or corrections officer or family member or previous arresting officer might be able to supply the presumptive ID.

Birthmarks come in many varieties. One distinctive type is called a port-wine stain (*nevus flammeus*). It is a reddish or purplish discoloration, and it may be small or cover a large area such as an entire shoulder or half of someone's face. Former Soviet President Mikhail Gorbachev had one on his forehead. They are typically very irregular, like an amoeba, and thus have a shape or pattern that is distinctive since no two are exactly alike. So if your suspect or corpse had such a mark, an old photo revealing the mark could be used to make a fairly positive ID.

As you know, many tattoos can be traced to the artist, especially today, since many are considered body art and some tattoo artists have distinctive techniques and loyal followings. Many tattooists use black pigments that contain carbon, reds that contain mercuric chloride, and greens that contain potassium dichromate. Others use aniline-based dyes. It is possible to extract some of the pigment from the corpse's skin and possibly exclude or confirm that a specific artist did the work.

Certain gangs boast their own tattoos. In California the CAL-GANG database stores such data, and often a query will result in a hit. This type of lead may result in the ultimate identification of the victim.

Can the Age of Surgical Scars Aid in Victim Identification?

Q: My protagonist is a detective who is confronted with a female corpse whose hands and head have been removed to hinder identification. She has a scar on her abdomen, which he believes is about three months old. This is important because a woman of about the same age and size was reported missing, and she had had her gallbladder removed three months before her disappearance. Can the age of scars be determined this accurately?

A: Yes and no. Any wound, whether surgical or from a knife fight, will follow the same healing pattern if it is closed properly with sutures and doesn't get infected. Lack of proper treatment or an infection of the wound would lead to delayed healing and more prominent scarring. Also, some people develop keloids when such wounds heal. A keloid is a raised thick scar that can be a half inch wide and rise a quarter inch above the surrounding tissue—sometimes more.

With normal healing the wound becomes mechanically strong after about two weeks. For several weeks the scar will be slightly pink to brownish red due to the microscopic blood vessels that invade the area to aid with the healing process. Over the next few months, as the body repairs the damage by laying down collagen (thick fibrous strands of connective tissue), the color gradually fades, and the scar shrinks considerably. With further maturing of the scar it finally becomes a faint white line by four to six months. The collagen continues to shrink until about one year. Thereafter, the scar remains unchanged for life. This means that the age of a scar can be approximated in the first four to six months, but after that all bets are off.

Your astute detective could see a 6-inch diagonally directed wound in the right upper quadrant of the corpse's abdomen and construe that it was from a cholecystectomy (gallbladder removal). He could further see that it appeared well healed but still possessed a pinkish hue and deduce that the wound was likely between six weeks and four months old. This would at least leave open the possibility that the missing woman and the corpse were one and the same. However, dental records, DNA evidence, or some other form of identification would be necessary to determine the true identity of the victim.

Will Stomach Contents Reveal When and What the Victim Ingested?

Q: My murder victim is found in the middle of the night. I have two questions. First, for a high-profile case, would the autopsy be done early the next morning? Second, can the autopsy tell very specifically what the victim ate? For example, if the victim ate chicken, vegetables, and bread five to six hours before death, would the contents still be visible at the time of the autopsy? Also, can the autopsy determine specific fluids and drugs, such as Coca-Cola versus tea or aspirin versus Alka-Seltzer? Would it be logical for a medical examiner to find traces of bicarbonate of soda and aspirin if the victim took Alka-Seltzer shortly before death?

A: Yes, the autopsy could be done the next morning. The M.E. could simply juggle the day's schedule and handle the high-profile case first. Also, in many jurisdictions the M.E.'s office has a "special cases room" where "special case" postmortem examinations can be videotaped.

Stomach and intestinal contents found at autopsy depend on

several factors such as the type and amount of foods consumed and the time lapse between ingestion and death. Digestive processes cease at death. Various foods remain in the stomach for different amounts of time. In general the stomach empties by four to six hours and the small intestines by twelve hours. If food material is found in the stomach, it would be reasonable for the M.E. to determine that death likely occurred within four hours of the meal. If the stomach is empty, he might conclude that the victim ate more than six hours before death.

Partially digested food, either in the stomach or in the small intestine, might reveal what that last meal was. This would be particularly true for high-cellulose foods such as corn since the body cannot digest cellulose. The vegetables in your scenario may still be identifiable, especially if you shorten the time between eating and death to less than four hours.

The stomach contents, blood, and urine would be tested for drugs. Unless death occurred shortly after ingestion, finding Coke or tea and distinguishing aspirin from Alka-Seltzer would be difficult.

Aspirin is acetylsalicylic acid (ASA), which is also in Alka-Seltzer (which also contains sodium bicarbonate and citric acid). Once ASA is in the bloodstream, it would be impossible to tell what ASA-containing product it came from unless undigested pills were present in the stomach. This is unlikely with Alka-Seltzer and aspirin since both dissolve readily.

Coke is simply sugar syrup, colorings and flavorings, caffeine, and carbonated water, all of which are digested and absorbed into the bloodstream fairly quickly. Most teas also contain caffeine.

Bicarbonate is a normal electrolyte in blood, so unless a large amount of Alka-Seltzer was ingested, it would be difficult to trace after digestion.

The M.E. could easily detect ASA, which is invariably part of a routine drug screen, and caffeine. Finding abnormal levels of bicarbonate would be more difficult and much less specific.

A complete examination of the crime scene could help the M.E.

here. If food was still on the table or in the refrigerator, it would help him analyze the stomach contents by narrowing his focus. The same would be true if aspirin and Alka-Seltzer bottles were found. The M.E. uses all the evidence he can accumulate, not just the autopsy, drug screen, and so forth, in making his assessment of cause and manner of death.

Can the Type of Alcohol Found in Stomach Contents Be Determined?

Q: In my story an old woman with a fondness for wine is found shortly after death in the tub of her stiflingly hot trailer. Would chemical analysis during an autopsy show what kind of alcohol the woman was drinking? Although she is known to drink only wine, a glass with a small amount of whiskey in it is found on the edge of the tub. Also, if distinctions between whiskey and wine can be detected, could an analysis also determine the brand of the whiskey? Would an autopsy show that the woman was actually drunk or only that she did indeed have alcohol in her system?

A: The M.E. might be able to determine the type of alcohol consumed if the victim expired shortly after drinking it. Since digestive processes cease at death, the stomach contents stay more or less intact. Decay and bacterial-mediated putrefaction would alter them over time, and these processes are accelerated in a warm environment. But this process might take a couple of days or more in most circumstances. If the stomach contents were well preserved, it might be possible to determine the type and even the brand of the alcohol.

If the alcohol was consumed a couple of hours or more before death, the digestive process would be fairly complete, since alcohol is basically a type of sugar and digests readily. The stomach contents probably would not be helpful, and once alcohol is in the bloodstream, it is alcohol. Blood analysis could distinguish ethanol (ethyl alcohol, the type in alcoholic beverages) from methanol (methyl alcohol, which is denatured alcohol, a poison) from isopropanol (isopropyl alcohol, which is rubbing alcohol), but if ethanol is found, it is generic ethanol; that is, in the bloodstream, wine is like vodka is like a good sour mash whiskey.

The blood alcohol level can be readily determined, and it is this level that dictates legal intoxication. In California the legal limit is 0.08 milligrams of alcohol per 100 milliliters of blood. This varies from state to state. Some people—and this seems more prevalent in women than in men—can become impaired at lower levels. Everyone is different. The M.E. could determine the blood alcohol level, and even if it was below the legal limit, he might be able to make a good guess as to the victim's level of impairment.

Can an Autopsy Reveal a History of Pregnancy or Childbirth?

Q: If a female corpse is autopsied soon after death, can the pathologist tell if she has had children or been pregnant? What if the body is partially decomposed from several months' exposure to cold weather?

A: After pregnancy there are permanent changes in the microscopic architecture of the breast and uterine tissues, which the M.E. would see. Also after pregnancy, pale striations often appear over the surface of the breasts and abdomen. These are similar in appearance to stretch marks and may have a faint pinkish, bluish, or silvery hue. Whether these tissue clues would help in your scenario depends on how well preserved the body is. The cold weather may help in this regard by delaying corpse putrefaction and decomposition.

Even in skeletonized remains, evidence of the trauma caused by previous childbirth is often present. Multiple pregnancies and deliveries make this evidence more profound. The M.E. would look for scars on the pubic bone that result from tears of the periosteum (the layer of tissue that covers the bones) and at the insertion sites of the various tendons that attach to the pelvic bones. It wouldn't be possible to determine how many children she had delivered, only that she had had at least one.

Can the Coroner Determine the Caliber of a Bullet by Simple Inspection?

Q: If an M.E. recovers a bullet during an autopsy, can he determine the millimeter gauge of the bullet, or would ballistics determine that?

A: Both. The M.E. could make a guess as to the type of bullet, but confirmation would require a true ballistics exam. Depending on how much damage the bullet suffered, an experienced M.E. could tell a .38 slug from a .45 from a 30.06, and some are very good at it. A complete ballistics evaluation would follow to confirm this and to make the information more acceptable in court.

In Slashing Wounds, Can the M.E. Determine What Weapon Was Used?

Q: I have a victim of a slashing being autopsied. How would I describe the wound if it is from a sharp claw versus a sharp instrument? How would the medical examiner know that the wound was caused by something other than a knife?

A: In general, slashing or cutting wounds are extremely difficult to analyze. Determining the type of weapon is virtually impossible. With stab wounds you have depth, width, thickness, angle of attack, shape of the blade, and sometimes serrations that help determine what type of weapon was used. These same characteristics make comparison with a suspected weapon easier.

With slashing wounds these characteristics don't exist. A Bowie knife and a dagger make very different stab wounds but similar slash wounds simply because the nature of the slashing motion produces a long wound with ragged edges that bleeds considerably.

A claw or talon could make a similar wound. The pathologist might be able to determine the width and at least a minimum length of the object by the depth and width of the wound, but little else unless trace evidence (fur, talon fragments, tissue, attacker's blood) was left behind.

Can the Coroner Distinguish Between Freshwater and Saltwater Drowning?

Q: In my story an elderly man with early-stage Alzheimer's is found floating in a bay, but he was actually drowned earlier in a backyard swimming pool. Would chlorine from the pool show up in the man's system during autopsy? Because the victim is initially presumed to have drowned in the bay, would the medical examiner expect to find debris, such as small bits of vegetation or the like, in his lungs? What would the M.E. be looking for in a drowning situation like this?

A: In drownings the M.E. can determine if it was freshwater or salt water and should be able to determine if the water contained chlorine. This freshwater versus salt water distinction was used in the movie *Chinatown*.

To understand the differences between freshwater and saltwater drownings, let's first take up the issue of osmosis. Osmosis is the passage of a liquid through a semipermeable membrane driven by a concentration gradient. Simple, huh? Let me explain. We use the term "tonicity" to describe the concentration of electrolytes (sodium, potassium, chloride, and so forth) in a liquid. The major electrolyte in the human body and in the blood is salt or sodium chloride (NaCl). "Isotonic" means the liquid has the same tonicity or NaCl concentration as blood. If the tonicity is less, as in fresh or pool water, it is termed hypotonic ("hypo" means lower or less). If the tonicity is higher, as in salt water, which contains a higher concentration of salt than blood, it is called hypertonic ("hyper" means above or more).

For our discussion a semipermeable membrane is a barrier that allows water to pass through but not other molecules such as sodium chloride. Water moves across this barrier from the hypotonic (lower concentration) liquid toward the hypertonic (higher concentration) liquid (Figure 19a). This movement continues until the tonicity on each side of the membrane is the same. In reality the water molecules continue to move back and forth, but once the tonicity is equal, the movement of water in each direction is equal. Think of it as the relatively hypertonic liquid acting like a sponge that "pulls" water toward it. Once things balance on each side of the membrane, this sponge effect is lost.

The tissues of the lungs are semipermeable membranes designed to allow oxygen and carbon dioxide free movement back and forth. The blood that bathes the lung tissue is isotonic.

In a freshwater drowning (Figure 19b), hypotonic fluid is introduced into the lungs. This causes water to move from the water-filled air sacs of the lungs into the bloodstream. This occurs because the isotonic blood is actually hypertonic relative to the hypotonic freshwater. This movement of water dilutes the blood,

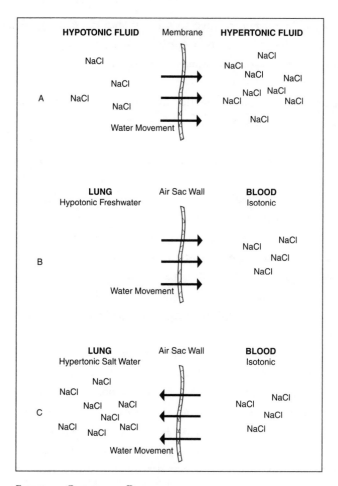

FIGURE 19. OSMOSIS AND DROWNING
Osmosis is the movement of water across a semipermeable membrane from a relatively hypotonic environment into a relatively hypertonic one (19a). In a freshwater drowning (19b), water moves from the air sacs of the lungs into the bloodstream, diluting the blood's sodium chloride content. A saltwater drowning (19c) results in movement of water from the relatively hypotonic bloodstream into the hypertonic salt-water-filled air sacs.

making it hypotonic relative to what it should be. In a saltwater drowning (Figure 19c), the opposite occurs. Salt water is hypertonic relative to blood, so water moves out of the bloodstream and into the air sacs of the lungs.

The M.E. would examine the lungs and the blood of the victim. In a freshwater drowning he would expect to see relatively dry air sacs (the water has moved into the bloodstream) and diluted or hypotonic blood. In a saltwater drowning he would expect to see wet air sacs (the water moves from the blood toward the salt-water-filled lung tissue) and concentrated or hypertonic blood. If he didn't find what was expected, he might conclude the body had been moved. It is important to note that this process of water movement doesn't happen instantly, so if the victim is pulled from the water quickly, little change may be detectable on these exams.

In your scenario the M.E. could find evidence for freshwater drowning and could find the lungs contained some residual chlorinated water. He would deduce that the victim had drowned in a swimming pool and not in a saltwater bay.

Yes, the victim's mouth, throat, and even his lungs could contain debris, vegetation, algae, and even small aquatic creatures, which would be those found in the area of drowning. There would be a mismatch if the body was moved to a different location after death. This was used in the film *Silence of the Lambs* when the larvae found in the throat of one victim was that of a rare moth that wasn't indigenous to the United States. The same can be said for vegetation. Of course, in a swimming pool the victim would probably not aspirate any vegetation or debris. If he drowned in a pond or lake, then freshwater vegetation or bugs rather than chlorine would be the findings that cause the M.E. concern. Here the M.E. would state that the victim was moved because the drowning was freshwater and the vegetation and bugs were freshwater life forms; thus, the victim could not have drowned in the saltwater bay.

Will an Autopsy Determine If Chlorine Is Present in the Lungs?

Q: I know the M.E. can determine whether a drowning is freshwater or salt water, but can chlorine be detected in a drowning victim and lead to the conclusion that the drowning occurred in a pool rather than a bathtub?

A: Yes. Samples of the lung tissue and any liquid that the lungs contain can be tested for chlorine. Some labs have to send the samples away to a more sophisticated lab for analysis, but the chlorine can be detected in most cases.

Do Skin and Nail Changes Occur with Some Poisons?

Q: I've read that some poisons can be determined by examining the skin and fingernails of the victim. Is this true? Do you have any examples of which poisons can be detected this way?

A: Yes. Many poisons cause changes in the skin, hair, mucous membranes of the mouth, and nails.

Lead: Chronic lead poisoning (plumbism) has been around for many centuries and may have led the decline of the Roman and Greek empires. Today it usually comes from exposure to lead-containing paints, gasoline, and plumbing pipes, and cooking or eating from ceramic containers that are finished with lead-containing glazes. Plumbism is associated with anemia, headache, abdominal pain, joint pain, fatigue, memory problems, neuropathies (weakness and/or numbness in an extremity), and a blue-black line at the junction of the teeth with the gums, called a "lead line."

Mercury: In children mercury poisoning can cause a syndrome known as acrodynia or pink disease. It is characterized by flushing, itching, swelling, excessive salivation and sweating, weakness, red, irregular skin rashes, and scaling of the skin on the palms and feet.

Arsenic: Chronic exposure to arsenic can cause hyperkeratosis and hyperpigmentation (thickening and darkening) of the skin, exfoliative dermatitis (flaking and sloughing of the skin), and transverse white lines in the fingernails, called Mee's Lines. Arsenic can be detected in the hair of victims of chronic poisoning.

Cyanide: Cyanide is a metabolic poison in that it blocks cytochrome oxidase, an enzyme found in the mitochondria of the cells. The mitochondria are responsible for cellular energy production and oxygen utilization. Blocking cytochrome oxidase prevents the cells from using oxygen, resulting in their death.

Cyanide forms cyanmethhemoglobin through a complex interaction with the hemoglobin found in the red blood cells, which lends a bright cherry red color to the blood. Because of this it can be confused with carbon monoxide poisoning (see below).

Hypostasis (lividity) is the postmortem settling of blood in dependent areas due to gravity. Typically, this is blue-gray or purple in color. With cyanide poisoning the cyanmethhemoglobin imparts a reddish hue to the settling blood so that dependent lividity in this situation takes on a brick red or dark pink color.

Carbon monoxide: Carbon monoxide combines with the hemoglobin in the red blood cells to form carboxyhemoglobin, which gives the blood and tissues a cherry red hue.

Is There a Poison That Can't Be Detected or That Can Be Masked by Venom?

Q: For my story, I need to know if there is a poison that either will not leave a forensics fingerprint or that can be covered by either scorpion venom or that of a rattlesnake.

A: Your best bet would be succinylcholine. It is an injectable muscular paralytic that paralyzes all muscles. The victim is awake and alert but can't move, speak, bat an eye, or breathe. Death is in about three or four minutes. The drug is quickly broken down in the body, so the M.E. is unlikely to find the drug even if he tests for it—with one exception.

If the injection site is visible, he could excise the tissue in the area and test it for the drug's breakdown products. As the drug is destroyed by the body's enzymes, it is converted to other compounds, and these compounds are called "breakdown products." Remnants of these substances would be left behind in the tissues near the point of injection. The famous case of Carl Coppolino's murder of his wife was solved using this technique. Coppolino was an anesthetist, so he had access to the drug. His wife's body was exhumed and the injection site located. Tissue testing gave the results needed to convict him.

If the M.E. found venom, a bite or sting site, and skin and blood changes that went along with the venom, he would assume that the cause of death was due to the venom. Looking for an injection site and testing for succinylcholine breakdown products would probably not be considered.

One caveat: The venom must be given while the victim is alive. Its local tissue destruction and its destructive effects on blood cells ceases at death when the circulation and all the body's metabolic processes stop. The M.E. would need to see the effects of the venom to conclude that it was the proximate cause of death. The victim could be paralyzed, maybe partially with a series of small doses of succinylcholine, and then exposed to the snake or scorpion. The victim would indeed die from the venom, but his death wouldn't be "accidental."

Succinylcholine can be found in hospital pharmacies, emergency rooms, and operating suites, so it could be stolen. Or it could be ordered from a pharmaceutical supplier.

Do Postmortem Wounds Bleed?

Q: If a person is murdered with a poison and then within a half hour a dagger is stuck into his throat to make it look as if the dagger was the cause of death, would the person bleed much?

A: I assume you mean the person was stabbed after death from the poison. In that case he would not bleed since the blood in the body clots fairly quickly once the action of the heart has ceased and the blood stagnates. The M.E. would be able to determine that the wound occurred after death in most cases.

If, on the other hand, the victim was stabbed when he was incapacitated by the poison but still alive, he would bleed, and the fact that he was also poisoned would have to await the M.E.'s toxicological studies.

What Do "Mood" Cosmetics Look Like on a Corpse?

Q: What would happen to "mood" cosmetics (lipstick and nail polish) that change color on live bodies with warm and cool temperatures after that person becomes a corpse?

A: Cosmetics are topical; that is, they sit on the surface of the lips and nails and do not interact with the tissues of the body. Thus, the product wouldn't know if the wearer was dead or alive. If the product actually interacted with the body's tissues, it would be designated a pharmaceutical agent, would come under FDA scrutiny, and wouldn't be classified as a cosmetic.

These "mood" products, predominantly lipstick and nail polish, react to heat. They change color over a specified range depending on the temperature. They are marketed to teenage girls because they "change colors with your body heat and mood." The color changes depend on the manufacturer and the particular product, but they tend to brighten as body temperature increases. I guess that way people can tell whether the wearer is "cool" or "hot."

Ranges include: purple to red, pastel blue to pink, and green gold to shimmering gold. You get the picture.

They would likely undergo their characteristic temperature-related color changes whether they were on a living person or a corpse. Of course, corpses tend to be cold, so the color range of the product would tend toward the cold end of its scale. However, if the body was found after several hours in a very warm room, because the corpse's temperature becomes that of the environment and these products reflect that temperature level, they would move toward their warmer range of color.

Cool idea, or is it hot? I never can keep those straight.

How Was Death Determined in the Seventeenth Century?

Q: I am working on a story set in seventeenth-century England. The uncle of my young female protagonist lapses into a coma from too much alcohol and opium, and is nearly buried alive. Her love interest, a doctor in training, discovers he is alive before the burial can take place. My question is, how was death determined during that time period?

A: Today we have sophisticated methods for determining death. Blood pressure, pulse, and respiration are examined, of course, but these can be inaccurate in certain circumstances. A person who overdoses on drugs, such as barbiturates, opium and its derivatives (heroin, morphine, and so forth), and tetraodontoxin (puffer fish toxin), to name a few, may appear dead. Their pulse may be so slow, their blood pressure so low, and their respirations so shallow that these vital signs may not be readily obtainable. This is particularly true if they are found in a cold environment where they are also cold to the touch and appear pale or blue-gray in color. An electrocardiogram (EKG) can determine if cardiac activity is present, and an electroencephalogram (EEG) can show brain activity. Death will be diagnosed if either is absent.

These technologies were not available three hundred years ago. Instead, tobacco smoke enemas, vigorous nipple pinching either manually or with pliers, hot pokers shoved into various bodily orifices, and aggressive tongue pulling were all used to determine if the corpse was truly dead. Tongue pulling was so popular that a device was developed that clamped the tongue and yanked it in and out when a crank was turned. This continued for several hours, and when the victim didn't complain, a pronouncement of death occurred. As you can guess, the occasional corpse rose from the dead during such procedures.

Many physicians of that era stated that the only true way to ascertain death was to await the appearance of putrefaction. Since families preferred not to have rotting corpses in the house, a system of "vitae dubiae asylums" or "waiting mortuaries" was established. The suspected dead person was placed in these institutions in a warm spot (to hasten the decomposition) until decay appeared, after which he could be buried. If he was indeed alive, he could signal this by pulling on a string, which was attached to a bell. Since corpses may manifest twitches and jerks from involuntary contractions of the decomposing muscles, false alarms were not uncommon. This was a disconcerting event to the person charged with overseeing the mortuary, I would suspect.

Another contraption available was the "security coffin." Again, the corpse could signal that he was indeed among the living by use of a bell, horn, or flag. And again, involuntary movements could cause false alarms.

Your young physician could pinch the uncle's nipples or yank on his tongue, or he could visit the mortuary and see a waving flag or hear a bell ringing and find the uncle now sober and very much alive.

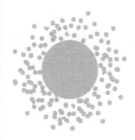

ODDS AND ENDS, MOSTLY ODDS

Do the Pupils Enlarge or Shrink with Death?

Q: I'm confused. Do the pupils enlarge or shrink at death?
Exactly when does this happen—before death, after, or
at the exact moment?

A: The pupils dilate (enlarge) at death. This makes the eyes of a
dead person appear black. The pupils dilate before death in most
cases. This occurs because the sympathetic nervous system (the
fight-or-flight part) is activated in any stressful situation, which
impending death would definitely fit. This activation causes release
of epinephrine (adrenaline) from the adrenal glands, which
increases blood pressure and heart rate as well as dilates the pupils.

At death the pupillary muscles relax, which also opens up the
pupils.

Do Bodies Move During Cremation?

Q: I have read that when a body is cremated using modern
techniques (crematorium), there is a tendency for the
body to sit up at some point due to the sudden contrac-

tion of the abdominal muscles. Is this true? Is it common, or does it happen only under certain conditions?

A: This may occur. More likely the body would assume the "pugilistic position." The legs draw up, the body hunches forward, and the arms flex so that the fists are beneath the chin, like a fighter. This happens when people die in fires and is due to muscular contraction that occurs as the heat evaporates water from the muscles. If this occurred in a cremation, it would be short-lived since the extreme heat used during cremation rapidly destroys the body.

How Is Body Weight Determined in a Quad Amputee?

Q: I write a fantasy series and have a recurring character who was born with no arms or legs, the result of a botched abortion that only succeeded in sucking his arms and legs off. From time to time he must be moved from his motorized chair to a car and back again by a female character. My question is, what would an adult male, without arms or legs, weigh?

A: Wild question.

Basically, the torso is about 50 percent of the body's weight, give or take a little. His weight would depend on his overall size and weight if he was "whole." If his normal weight would be 150 pounds, then 75 to 80 is good. If he were a big man—say 200 pounds—then 100, and so on.

If he has a portion of his shoulders and upper arms, add another 10 percent and if he has a portion of his thighs, add another 15 percent. If his amputations are at the joints, which I suspect is the case from your description, use the 50 percent number, and you'll be in the ballpark.

What Drug Is Used for Animal Euthanasia?

Q: I am working on a story in which a child's pet dog is critically injured and must be put down. What drug is used? Is it injected? How long does the dog take to die? Would the dog feel anything? Would the veterinarian do this procedure alone, or would he have an assistant with him?

A: There are several manufacturers of veterinary euthanasia products. One of the commonly used ones is Eutha-6, or Euthanol. Its active components are pentobarbital (a barbiturate sedative) and alcohol. A large dose is given so that the animal basically dies from a barbiturate and alcohol overdose.

An IV is started in the animal's forepaw. The leg is shaved and the IV is placed in a vein and taped down. This would be the only discomfort involved. The dose is then given, and the dog goes to sleep in a matter of seconds, perhaps five to ten. Breathing ceases almost as quickly. The heart might take three to four minutes to stop, but all in all it is a quick and painless procedure.

The vet typically has an assistant with him to help hold and comfort the dog, start the IV, give the injection, and/or comfort the owners if they chose to be present. He could do it by himself, but most often there are two people involved.

Will Oleander Poison a Cat?

Q: I need to have a cat poisoned (fictionally, of course) with something that makes him quite ill until he upchucks, after which he recovers. Any suggestions as to what to use? My poisoner has used oleander to kill one human. Could he use oleander on a cat, with the cat surviving?

A: Oleander *(Nerium oleander)* would work well here since its toxicity is dose dependent. That means a small amount will make you sick and a larger amount will kill you, unlike cyanide, where almost any amount will kill you.

Many dogs and cats and children have died or become ill from eating oleander leaves, flowers, and so forth (all parts of the plant are poisonous). Have the poisoner give the cat a very small amount, and he will get sick but survive. The actual amount? I have no idea. Just have him crush up a single leaf or flower and feed it to the cat in some food or meat. That should do it.

What "Hot" Substance Can Be Used to Sabotage Someone's Diaphragm?

Q: I have an unusual question. A teenage girl catches her dad having an affair with a young mother whose child the teenager baby-sits. She wants to punish the young mom and her dad. Could something be put on the woman's diaphragm that would cause them some discomfort? I thought of Vicks VapoRub or Ben-Gay, but these would be detectable before she inserted it. Any other ideas?

A: Tabasco. No contest. It could be applied and allowed to dry, after which it would have little if any odor and wouldn't be visible or change the feel of the diaphragm. But add a little moisture, and she'll get the message immediately. If she also uses a spermicidal jelly, that might delay the onset of symptoms by diluting the Tabasco slightly and by coating the vaginal lining. Once intercourse begins, however, the Tabasco would begin to irritate these tender tissues and perhaps the man's also. First a little tingle and a little heat, then more tingle and burn, and finally severe burning and panic. What a totally diabolical question.

Do Blind People Have "Visual" Dreams?

Q: In my story a seven-year-old boy who has been blind since birth begins experiencing vivid and frightening dreams. Do the blind "see" people and objects in their dreams?

A: Blind individuals can be considered in two broad categories. Congenitally blind persons are sightless from birth, while adventitiously blind persons lose their sight at some later time. Children who are blind before age five or so tend to have much in common with those who are congenitally blind. Since their blindness began at such an early age, they possess little memory of images and colors and thus are less able to "see" things compared with those who became blind after age seven. This lack of imagery spills over into their dreams.

Many researchers in this area consider dreaming a constructive cognitive process; that is, we construct our dream worlds based on our sensory experiences. What we see, hear, feel, smell, and taste contributes to the building of our dreams.

Most congenitally blind people are able to "see" spatial relationships in their dream constructs, and some can even create visual forms, but they do not see the actual objects. What they see in their dreams tends to parallel what they see in their waking lives. Some are able to construct at least amorphous images better than others. Those who become blind later in life tend to have dream visualizations that parallel the waking visual experiences they had before they became blind.

The congenitally blind and those who become adventitiously

blind before age five may have vivid and detailed dreams, but they do not see images of people or structures or objects. They tend to feel the same emotions and have similar reactions to nightmares, but their dreams are more amorphous.

Those who become blind between ages five and seven may or may not see images. It depends on the individual.

Interestingly, many people who become blind after age seven have visually detailed dreams forever, while others do so for only twenty to thirty years. It is as if their memories of images fade and thus the images also fade from their dreams.

Your character would not see images but could still have very emotional dreams and frightening nightmares. He would describe his dream experiences in terms of feelings and sounds and smells, which can be even more frightening than visions, but the images would be vague and poorly defined. As with all of us, what he experiences will reflect the things that occur in his waking life. His problems, fears, wants, interests, conflicts, preoccupations, attitudes, and fantasies will play out in his dream world.

A FEW FINAL WORDS

Now that you have completed your journey through this book, I hope that you writers and readers have learned something from each and every question and answer. Some were simple and straightforward; others were complex and sophisticated; and still others were downright bizarre.

Yet each question reveals the incredible imagination, curiosity, and dedication to getting it right that is essential for credible storytelling and fiction writing. I believe these questions provide insight into the creative process and demonstrate the depth of commitment to craft that is found in successful writers of fiction.

I hope you found these pages interesting, informative, and stimulating. It is my sincerest wish that this information will improve your own writing and reading and stir your creative literary juices.

Thank you for your time, interest, and curiosity.

Visit Dr. Lyle's Web site, The Writers Medical and Forensics Lab, at www.dplylemd.com.

ABOUT THE AUTHOR

D. P. Lyle, M.D., writes "The Doctor Is In," a monthly medical and forensic Q&A column for *The March of Crime* and *The Sleuth Sayer,* two newsletters for the Mystery Writers of America (Southern California and Southwestern chapters). He has practiced cardiology in Orange County, California, for the past twenty-five years.